A BREAKTHROUGH PLAN

FROM THE EDITORS OF **Prevention**®

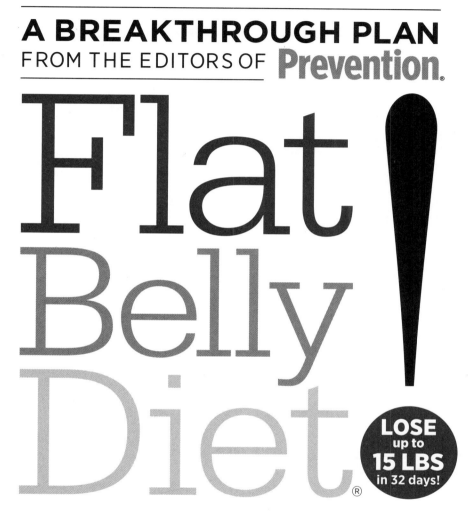

Flat Belly Diet!

LOSE
up to
15 LBS
in 32 days!

A FLAT BELLY IS ABOUT FOOD & ATTITUDE. PERIOD. (NOT A SINGLE CRUNCH REQUIRED)

BY LIZ VACCARIELLO, Editor-in-Chief, with Cynthia Sass, MPH, RD

RODALE®

Direct and trade editions are both being published in 2008.

Direct edition photo credits: Back cover photographs (bottom left) by Kristine Larsen; (top right) by Marcus Nilsson, food styling by Anne Disrude, prop styling by Deborah Williams for Pat Bates and Associates; (tape measure photo) by Ted Morrison

Trade edition photo credits: Tape measure photo by Ted Morrison.

Cover and interior design by Jill Armus

Interior exercise photos © Tom MacDonald/Rodale Images
Before/after/now photos by Kristine Larsen

Library of Congress Cataloging-in-Publication Data

Flat belly diet! : a flat belly is about food & attitude, period. (not a single crunch required) / by Liz Vaccariello, editor-in-chief ; with Cynthia Sass. — Rev. ed.
    p.   cm.
    Includes bibliographical references and index.
    ISBN-13: 978-1-60529-959-4 (direct hardcover)
    ISBN-10: 1-60529-959-6 (direct hardcover)
    ISBN-13: 978-1-59486-851-1 (trade hardcover)
    ISBN-10: 1-59486-851-4 (trade hardcover)
    1. Reducing diets. 2. Abdomen. I. Vaccariello, Liz. II. Sass, Cynthia.
RM222.2.F535 2008a
613.2'5—dc22   2008010908

Distributed to the trade by Macmillan

4 6 8 10 9 7 5   direct hardcover
2 4 6 8 10 9 7 5 3   trade hardcover

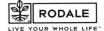

RODALE
LIVE YOUR WHOLE LIFE™

We inspire and enable people to improve their lives and the world around them

For more of our products visit **rodalestore.com** or call 800-848-4735

FOR THE MILLIONS WHO BEMOAN

THEIR BELLIES, SO THEY CAN

LEARN TO LOVE THEM INSTEAD.

—Liz and Cynthia

contents

acknowle

dgments

We dedicate the *Flat Belly Diet* to the readers of *Prevention*—all 11 million of you—who have told us in no uncertain terms that belly fat is your biggest physical challenge.

Our gratitude to the Rodale family. For generations, through their magazines, books, and online properties, they have been committed to a special mission, that of giving people the tools and inspiration to live their whole lives. Our most heartfelt thanks to Rodale CEO Steve Murphy, whose leadership means Rodale is the kind of company where creativity is nurtured and the highest standards are set—and met—daily. It all starts with the edit, Steve!

Like magazines, books are a collaborative effort, and this one is no exception. Very special thanks to Gregg Michaelson ("Let's make it happen!"), Janine Slaughter, Liz Perl Erichsen, and Jim Berra (the unsung hero behind all things *Prevention*). To Robin Shallow, who never met an idea she didn't improve, and Karen Mazzotta, who is tireless in her enthusiasm, support, and belief in this plan. And to Fotoulla Euripidou, for her understanding of the *Prevention* audience and for helping us determine whether *Prevention* readers would be interested in this kind of diet book—by asking them!

We'd also like to extend our gratitude to the original members of our initial test panel, which was conducted in summer of 2007. They first opened our eyes to how special the *Flat Belly Diet* really was. Thank you Mary Aquilar, Syndi Becker, Katherine Brechner, Donna Christiano, Evelyn Gomer, Diane Kaspareck, Patti Lloyd, Kevin Martin, Nichole Michl, Colleen O'Neill-Groves, Julie Plavsic, and Mary Anne Speshok for devoting your summer to this project and providing us with the essential insights that helped us develop this book beyond daily meal plans. Thank you also Gina Allchin, President, Health Trek P.T.T., who measured each and every one of our panelists with precision and compassion—a tough combination!

You literally would not be holding this book in your hands without executive editor Nancy Hancock ("good to great!"). All thanks to her dedicated team, including Chris Krogermeier, Marina Padakis, Anthony Serge, JoAnn Brader, Keith Biery, Hope Clarke, Wendy Gable, and Ana Palmiero. And of course, to Ina Yalof—one of the fastest, most creative writers we've ever known—we offer a round of applause.

Big hugs to *Prevention*'s brilliant creative director, Jill Armus, whose ability to communicate elegance, authority, and strength through color and design have infused the entire *Prevention* brand of products (most recently this book cover and interior) with new vitality. And to *Prevention* fitness director Michele Stanten, whose contribution to and extensive review of Chapter 10 have helped make it one of the most authoritative sources of information on banishing belly fat with exercise.

Thanks also to Miriam Backes, Merritt Watts, Amy Gorin, Katie Kackenmeister, and Kristen Watson, who assisted with coordinating the test panel and editing and fact-checking the manuscript, even during precious nights and weekends. To Lori Conte, Courtenay Smith, and Polly Chevalier: for keeping the trains running on time. And to the smartest photo and art team in the business, including *Prevention*'s Helen Cannavale, Kim Latza, Faith Enemark, Jessica Sokol, and Donna Agajanian. And of course to Rosalie Rung, who helped capture the enormous success of our test panelists on film and video.

Our deepest gratitude we save for brand editor Leah McLaughlin, a longtime colleague and friend to both of us. From helping develop the initial idea to making sure the most engaging, authoritative manuscript shipped to the printer and every moment in between, Leah was critical to the launch of this book—not to mention the companion online subscription service, flatbellydiet.com.

Finally, we'd like to thank our husbands, Steve Vaccariello and Jack Bremen, and families (especially Olivia and Sophia Vaccariello and Diane Salvagno!) for putting up with all the late—late!—nights and never-ending conversations about *Flat Belly Diet* this and *Flat Belly Diet* that. (Yes, now we can take a weekend off, guys!)

GET READY FOR A FLAT BELLY

IT DOESN'T MATTER what your personal stumbling blocks are: baby weight, killer cravings, or (say it with me) "getting older." Belly fat is *not* your destiny. I am delighted to tell you that you can, and will, get rid of it. *Prevention* has found a way to target belly fat that is healthy, real, long-lasting, and works for everyone.

Before we get started, I think it's important to do a "gut check." Chances are, if you've plunked down cold, hard cash for a book called *Flat Belly Diet*, you may wish you had someone else's belly or wish you had your own belly—from 20 years ago.

If that's you, I ask you to change your thinking. Be kind to your belly. No matter how flat or round, jiggly or rock hard—it's yours, and it's powerful. It's probably the center of some of your most profound memories. Think about it . . . the laughter you've shared, the romantic dinners you've had, the butterflies you've felt, the children you may have carried. All these set up house in—yes—your belly. And for that it deserves your respect. Your appreciation. And more than a little love and kindness . . . even when you're struggling to button your jeans.

HOW DO I FEEL ABOUT MY BELLY? I consider it my core strength, and I love to feel it move, twist, support me as I go through life's business. It's where food (one of life's greatest pleasures, yes?) touches down, and there are few things as peaceful for me as that not-stuffed-not-hungry-but-just-full feeling. It's also my meditative center, and I sense the calm over-taking me when I fill my middle with deep breaths. Then, of course, there's the role it played in my pregnancy with twins. Anything willing to expand to host two precious, growing, kicking girls earns a special place in my heart for all time.

But the belly betrays. If I'm puffy the morning after a sushi dinner, that's where my outfit feels tight. If PMS strikes, my belly moans and groans. When I gain 5 pounds, that's where it shows. And, of course, when I go to take those 5 pounds off, that's where they stay.

One of the best things about being editor-in-chief of *Prevention* is hearing from all of you and learning—clearly and quickly—that I am not alone in my love/hate affair with this fascinating, troublesome part of the body. Many of you have told me that when look at yourself in the mirror, you overlook your familiar, beautiful features, the favorite nuances of your physique. Instead, your eye travels directly to the areas where your fat resides. And for most of us, that's the belly.

For countless reasons that I will outline throughout this book, the belly starts letting us down around age 40. Sometime between our 35th and 55th birthdays (some earlier, some later, and some, God willing, never), the belly pooches, puffs, and starts spilling over our waistbands. First we suck it in, yet it refuses to achieve its formerly flat shape. Then we crunch until our necks scream, while the fat over the sculpted abs muscles remains. And eventually we diet, then watch with frustration as the weight disappears from our breasts and our faces and the belly fat stays put. Eventually, belly fat starts to feel like our destiny—something that even hours on the treadmill or the strictest diet in the world won't budge. . . .

Until now.

MY QUEST TO FIND THE ABSOLUTE BEST WAY to blast belly fat started when I hired *Prevention*'s nutrition director, Cynthia Sass, MPH, RD. Her first challenge was to comb the latest research, combine it with her vast clinical experience, and develop a diet that would target abdominal fat specifically. I made a good decision—Cynthia is not only a phenomenal magazine editor but also a registered dietitian with two graduate degrees and 15 years of experience, including countless hours of working with women in the real world. And here's the best part: She is passionate about food! I knew that any diet I asked her to construct would be satisfying and delicious, that it would be a way of eating that women could embrace for a lifetime. And boy, was I right.

· She has developed a belly-shrinking eating plan that is grounded in the latest and most credible science (that you won't find anywhere else!)—and offers the most filling, satisfying, and delicious meals that you will ever have the pleasure of eating.

But my vision for this *Flat Belly Diet* went beyond food. I know that any successful diet acknowledges that we eat for emotional reasons as well as physical ones. Not only does the *Flat Belly Diet* deliver a healthy, satisfying way of eating—one that will rid your body of fat in the place you told us you want to slim down most—but it will teach you how to *want* to eat this way forever. The mental tricks, tips, and strategies are culled from the latest research and are designed to inspire you, motivate you, and set you up for a better relationship with food for the rest of your life!

Belly Fat Defined

WHEN I TOSS AROUND the words "belly fat," I'm actually talking about two different types: *subcutaneous* and *visceral*. **Subcutaneous fat** is best, though perhaps not most scientifically, defined as the fat that you can see, the "inch you can pinch." *Subcutaneous* means "beneath" (*sub*) "the skin" (*cutaneous*), and it's no big secret that this fat resides all over. In some spots—your thighs, underarms, *tummy, anyone?*—it may be thicker than in others, but for the most part it's everywhere, even on the soles of your feet. A moderate amount of subcutaneous fat is essential for life—for one thing, it keeps you from freezing to death in the winter. But too much of it causes dissatisfaction with how we look (which studies show leads to even more dangerous health behaviors). And worse: Excessive amounts of subcutaneous fat function as a visible sign of being overweight or obese, which doctors know raises your risk for many diseases. But I have some great news: Subcutaneous fat responds immediately to this diet plan.

Before you happily skip pages and move to the diet, let's talk about the second type of fat—visceral—which is much more dangerous and difficult to lose. **Visceral fat** resides deep within your torso and is sometimes referred to as "hidden" belly fat. I prefer the term "deadly." Because of its proximity to your heart and liver, excess visceral fat can increase your risk of all sorts of diseases, from heart disease and diabetes to cancer and Alzheimer's disease. And the most frustrating part? You can cut calories and exercise religiously and still be left with too much of it.

In fact, the only way to minimize both visceral and subcutaneous fat simultaneously is to eat the right . . . fat.

The New Belly-Flattening Nutrient

AT *PREVENTION*, we've been talking about the healthfulness of monounsaturated fat—the kind found in olive oil, nuts, and avocados—for decades. Nearly every issue contains some tip or strategy for getting more in your diet. In fact, we're on such intimate terms with monounsaturated fatty acids that we have a nickname for them—MUFAs (pronounced MOO-fahs). But it wasn't until the spring of 2007 that we realized just how amazing these fats are. That was when Spanish researchers published a study in the journal *Diabetes Care* showing that eating a diet rich in MUFAs *can actually help prevent weight gain in your belly.*[1]

The researchers looked at the effect of three different diets—one high in saturated fat, another high in carbohydrates, and a third rich in MUFAs—on a group of patients with "abdominal fat distribution," or, in language the rest of us nonscientists can understand, belly fat. All three diets contained the same number of calories, but only the MUFA diet was found to reduce the accumulation of belly fat and, more specifically, visceral belly fat.

Bear in mind: *No other nutrient can do this.* And that's what makes the *Flat Belly Diet* unlike any other diet book you've ever read. It presents the only diet to give MUFAs center stage, to make them an essential part of every single meal. And that means it's the only diet that helps you lose fat in the belly *specifically*! In Chapter 3, you'll read more about MUFAs and their various health benefits, but until then, let's take a broader look at this truly groundbreaking diet plan.

The Flat Belly Diet Program

THE FLAT BELLY DIET is made up of two parts—the *Four-Day Anti-Bloat Jumpstart* and the *Four-Week Eating Plan.* The whole thing together takes just 32 days, which studies show is just enough time to make any dietary change a lifestyle. Then, after you've mastered the program and seen the desired changes in your weight and measurements, I give you the tools to keep your belly flat for life. Even though you may be tempted to follow one part without the other, I want you to start with the Anti-Bloat Jumpstart, then move straight into the Four-Week Eating Plan. Here's why.

▧ THE FOUR-DAY ANTI-BLOAT JUMPSTART isn't just about beating bloat; it's also extremely important in sparking your emotional commitment to the entire program. The 4-day plan includes a prescribed list of foods and drinks that will help flush out fluid, reduce water retention, and relieve digestive issues like gas and constipation, which can make your belly puff unnecessarily. You'll drink Cynthia's signature Sassy Water and eat healthy foods like fruits, vegetables, and whole grains. When we tested this diet on our group of volunteers, one of the participants lost an amazing *7 pounds and 5 inches in the first 4 days (that's just 96 hours)*.

Losing the bloat isn't just a way to fit into your favorite dress again. It's about feeling confident, powerful, and proud of your body. Dropping even a few pounds of unnecessary water weight can be thrilling and can give you a major confidence boost—essential for success on any diet plan. Plus, I've added a second element to the 4-day plan: a Mind Trick at every meal. These quick and easy healthy-eating triggers will serve as mealtime reminders that you have embarked on a new way of life—a new way of living with and caring for your body.

What about Exercise?

I exercise every day, walking 50 minutes as part of my commute. (I also strength-train every weekend and try to fit in a weekly Pilates class or yoga session, too.) And I encourage everyone to make exercise a part of his or her lifestyle.

To that end, I asked *Prevention's* fitness director, Michele Stanten, to devise the exercise program in Chapter 10 for you to follow as you embark on the *Flat Belly Diet*. Adding a fitness program to the eating plan and mental strategies will mean faster results (it certainly did for some of our testers).

But what makes the *Flat Belly Diet* truly special is that *you don't need to exercise to reap the benefits*. If you do exercise, you will most certainly see results faster, and you

■ THE FOUR-WEEK EATING PLAN begins the morning after you complete the Anti-Bloat Jumpstart, and it's the centerpiece of this book. Every day you'll enjoy three supersatisfying 400-calorie meals and one 400-calorie Snack Pack. Each meal and snack contains just the right amount of MUFA to make that belly fat disappear. How simple is that? No calorie counting. No math! We chose the quantity of 1,600 calories per day because that's the precise amount an adult woman of average height, frame, size, and activity level needs to get down to her ideal body weight while maintaining a high energy level, healthy immune system, and strong muscles. It also ensures you won't feel tired, cranky, irritable, moody, or hungry.

But because no plan fits all, we've provided two different versions: The first one's perfect for people who have little time to spend in the kitchen. In Chapter 7, you'll find 84 different 400-calorie, MUFA-packed Quick-Fix Meals and 28 different 400-calorie Snack Pack options. Choose three meals and one Snack Pack a day and you're done. In a month, you'll have a flatter belly and I'll have done my job.

Sometimes, however, you'll want a more involved home-cooked meal, whether it's family night, or the weekend, or you're just a good cook who likes to flex her

will gain secondary benefits like improved cardiovascular health and stronger, more toned muscles. But you can still expect to shrink your belly—and lose both subcutaneous and visceral fat—by simply following the eating plan.

If you do not already exercise regularly, you don't have to start doing so right away. I have always been a big believer in the phrase "small changes, big results." To me, it's more important that you do *something* to reduce your belly fat than it is to do *everything,* only to find that too many changes are too overwhelming to maintain. If you do not already have a workout routine, incorporating a new way of eating into your lifestyle may be change enough for the first 32 days.

culinary muscles now and then. In Chapter 8, you'll find more than 80 recipes that all provide the requisite number of calories and MUFAs per serving, so they can be swapped in for any of your required three meals a day.

Like the Four-Day Anti-Bloat Jumpstart, the Four-Week Plan isn't only about what you eat. It's about how you think. In Chapter 9, I'll ask you to keep a daily journal—a key predictor of success on any diet. Every day, I'll prompt you to reflect on a particular aspect of your relationship to food, your belly, your body, and your goals. I call these reflections *Core Confidences*—not only because your belly lies at the physical center, or core, of your body, but also because your attitude is at the core of your ability to succeed . . . at anything.

Throughout this book, look for the boxes titled **Did You Know?** to learn more about fat, weight loss, and general health. These are quick tips, strategies, and bits of information that experts and readers tell me are useful. And don't forget to read the entries titled **Sass from Sass.** Cynthia wrote these to share her thoughts and advice about how to achieve success on this amazing program. You'll also find incredible success stories from the women (and men) who participated in our *Flat Belly Diet* test panel—and who have a flatter belly to prove it!

If I know one thing for certain after years editing *Prevention*, it's that maintaining a healthy mind and body are the absolute most important things I can do for myself—and my family. I hope that by the time you finish reading this book and following this plan, you will have fallen in love with your flatter belly, your healthier, wholesome way of eating, and the amazing energy and vitality that comes with better health!

Flat Belly Diet!

> The Four-Day Anti-Bloat Jumpstart

A full 96 hours is all it takes to spark your commitment to the *Flat Belly Diet*—and lose a few pounds! The Jumpstart consists of:

A DAILY DOSE OF SASSY WATER Created by Cynthia, this make-ahead concoction helps guard against dehydration.

A MIND TRICK AT EVERY MEAL Fast mental fixes help get your brain in the *Flat Belly* game.

> The Four-Week Plan

Twenty-eight days of delicious MUFA-packed meals and recipes that you can mix and match. The plan consists of:

FOUR 400-CALORIE MEALS A DAY Choose from our meal selections or recipes, and be sure to make one meal a Snack Pack.

A MUFA AT EVERY MEAL These superhealthy fats keep you feeling full and ensure every meal is exceptionally tasty.

ONE DAILY CORE CONFIDENCE REFLECTION Spend 15 minutes a day exploring your relationship to food and desire to reach your goals.

> An Optional Exercise Program

Fat-burning walks, a Metabolism Boost, and a Belly Routine will help you build muscle and maximize calorie burn.

READ A FLAT BELLY
SUCCESS
STORY

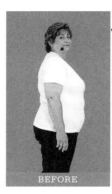

BEFORE

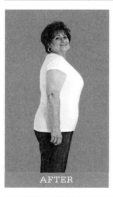

AFTER

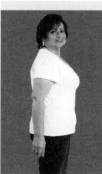

Mary Anne Speshok

AGE: 55

POUNDS LOST:

15

IN 32 DAYS

ALL-OVER
INCHES LOST:

10

At press time:

49

POUNDS
LOST
IN 5
MONTHS!

I'M NOT A KID ANYMORE," says 55-year-old Mary Anne Speshok. But you'd never know it from listening to her describe the effect of her new weight loss on her husband of 5 years. "He's chasing me around the room! Like I'm his toy! He looks at me and says, 'Wow! I can't believe what I'm seeing!'"

Mary Ann says her husband was as happy as she is with her results from the first 4 weeks on the *Flat Belly Diet*. In just 32 days, she had lost $3\frac{1}{2}$ inches off her hips, $3\frac{1}{2}$ off her stomach, 3 inches off her back—(that little place that hangs over the bra strap), and an inch on each thigh. "On the scale today, I lost 2 more pounds. I feel as if the weight is melting off of me. People tell me I'm walking with more confidence in my step. It's terrific!"

The administrative assistant has a message for anyone considering the *Flat Belly Diet*: "The only thing you have to do is start it. All the tools are there."

She calls it a revolutionary, doable winner—doable, she says, because the MUFAs keep you satisfied. "Most people, including me, don't stay with a diet plan because they get hungry between meals. The difference with this diet is you literally don't get hunger pains. It's revolutionary because you start seeing results so fast that you want to keep going." And the winner part? "Well," she adds, "just look at what I've lost."

Mary Anne has committed herself to doing the *Flat Belly* Workout in Chapter 10 along with the diet. Even though she works full-time and commutes an hour each way to and from work, she still manages to get in her paces. She usually walks 30 minutes at lunchtime, but on days when she can't, she stops at the gym even before she goes home and does her 30 minutes of walking there. At home, she either does floor exercises or uses hand weights. She says her energy level is so high these days that exercising is easy.

And like so many recently thin women, Mary Anne has just discovered how great it is to fit into a nice, slim pair of jeans. "I never even owned a pair before," she says. "I liked them, but just not on me." Not anymore, though. She says she just went out and bought three different styles of jeans because they all looked so good on her.

In fact, Mary Anne's closet is getting a full workout these days. She's buying new clothes to fit her new body. And she's adding bracelets and necklaces, "which I love. When I felt so big, I just wore my wedding ring and my watch. You don't want to call attention to yourself because you don't feel pretty. But now, bring on the jewelry! The more the better!" She and her husband are renewing their vows soon, and she's looking forward to wearing a beautiful gown that she hasn't been able to fit into for a long time. "What a prize for reaching your goal," she exclaims. "To fit into something that sat in your closet, just waiting. This beautiful gown . . . and a size smaller."

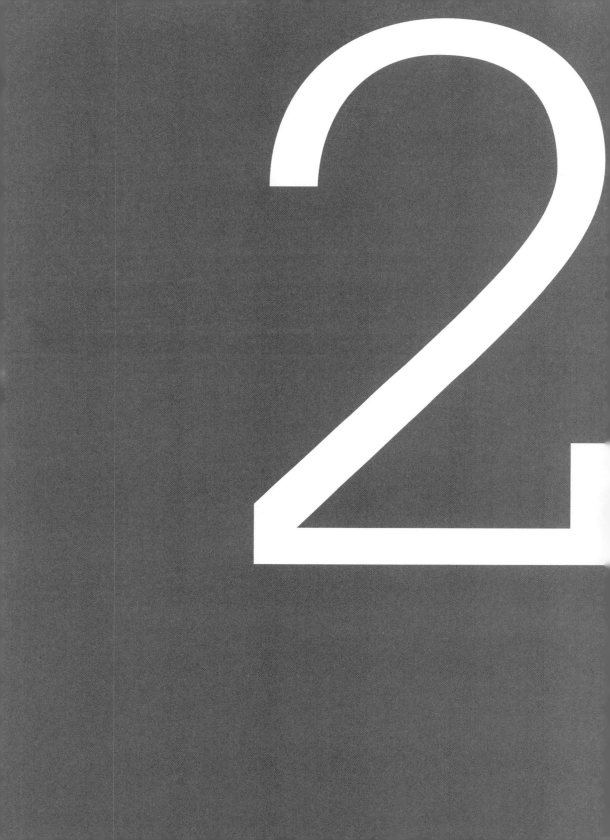

THE SKINNY ON BELLY FAT

BODY FAT IS ESSENTIAL. **Without it, you couldn't survive. Your cells wouldn't be able to hold together or absorb nutrients from the food you ate. Your organs wouldn't be able to produce the hormones that make you distinctly female. You would freeze to death on a cold day. You'd run the risk of damaging your internal organs just by bumping into a doorknob. And forget ever finding your keys again. Without fat, your brain probably wouldn't even be able to figure out what a key is.**

In effect, *you* wouldn't be *you* without fat. Body fat, whether it's found on your thighs or buttocks or within the intricate coils of your brain, plays a role in nearly every single biological function in your body, and it's impossible to live without it. Of course, there's a fine line between having just the right amount of body fat and having too much.

The Trouble with Belly Fat

SCIENTISTS HAVE KNOWN for some time now that excess body fat isn't good for you. Obesity—which, technically speaking, means "overfat"—is considered as deadly as smoking, according to some analyses. When you step on a scale, you're getting a rough indication of how heavy you are, but you can't tell how fat you are. The body mass index (BMI) gets you closer to figuring it out. Here's how to calculate it.

- Multiply your weight in pounds by 703.
- Divide that number by your height in inches.
- Divide that number by your height in inches again.

A woman who weighs 145 pounds and is 67 inches tall (5'7") has a BMI of 22.7. A woman who weighs 260 pounds and is 67 inches tall has a BMI of 40.7. You can also visit the BMI calculator at **flatbellydiet.com** for an instant calculation.

If your BMI is 25 or higher, you're considered "overweight," but if your BMI is 30 or above, you're "obese." If it's 40 or above, you're "morbidly obese," and your health is at great risk. A BMI below 18.5 is "underweight"—that's also cause for concern, because it indicates too low a percentage of body fat to ensure healthy functioning. An index between 18.5 and 24.9 is just right.

However, one of the problems with the body mass index is that it doesn't account for your muscle mass. As a result, some athletes—who have a much lower percentage of body fat and higher percentage of muscle—can compute to be overweight or, in some rare cases, obese.

More recently, studies have begun to show that while being obese in general is unhealthy, carrying excess body fat specifically *around your belly* is really, really unhealthy. Studies show that women who have waistlines measuring 35 inches or more are at greater risk for heart disease and diabetes than those whose waistline measurements are smaller. For men, a waistline measurement of 40 or above can be an indicator of the same health risks. Heart disease is the number one killer of American women, and rates of diabetes have reached epidemic levels. The connection between the measurement of your waist and your risk of dying from one of these diseases is no mere coincidence.

According to a study reported in the *New England Journal of Medicine,* people with large hips and small waists produce higher levels of HDL cholesterol, the protective form, than do those with large bellies.[1] (I like to remember the two types of cholesterol in this way: **H**DL is the "**h**ealthy" kind, **L**DL is the "**l**ousy" kind.) Women typically have higher HDL levels—which is linked to fewer heart attacks—than men do. But that all changes after menopause, when body fat distribution changes due to hormone shifts and a woman's risk for heart attack increases.

If you're overweight or obese, take your pick of things to blame—Alfredo sauce, for one. Not to mention ice cream and soda, and cake and cheese and—well, you get the picture. Eating too much of any food can make you fat. Cutting back on cardiovascular exercise is another way to add inches all over, as is skipping a strength-training routine. And for some of us, genetics plays a role. But something happens to us after age 40 that makes it easier to put on *belly fat* in particular: Our hormones go haywire.

As estrogen levels decline, your body struggles to maintain its hormonal

DID YOU KNOW?

We're all born with the same number of fat cells (about 40 billion, give or take). As we grow up, the number of fat cells we have increases until after our pubescent and adolescent years, when they are pretty much set. In the past, it was assumed that the only difference between overweight people and thin ones was that overweight or obese people had all their fat cells filled to maximum capacity. It's now known that we can—and do, in fact—"grow" more fat cells in adulthood. This is because when fat cells expand to their maximum size, they divide and increase again the number of fat cells. Some obese people have more fat cells than nonobese people. **But in the end, both the number and the size of the fat cells determine the amount of fat someone has.**

balance. In the process, body fat—which is extremely important in manufacturing estrogen and other sex hormones, not to mention preserving bone mass—becomes more valuable and thus harder to get rid of. As you enter perimenopause and hit menopause, your body fat distribution starts to look more like a man's and less like a woman's.

What do I mean by that? Well, you've heard of the term *beer belly*? Male body fat tends to concentrate around the belly area—and it doesn't really have much to do with beer, except for the fact that, because beer is a source of excess calories, it's generally a catalyst for weight gain. Female body fat, on the other hand, tends to concentrate around the hips, thighs, and butt during the years that we're most likely to reproduce. Some researchers theorize that as estrogen levels decline, a woman's body stops laying down fat in these trouble zones and starts laying down fat near the belly, like a man's body does.

Not every woman ends up with excess midsection weight in midlife. Although some women with small waists and large hips can with time develop a midsection large enough that it becomes the broadest part of her body, other women keep the "pear" shape forever. For them, the weight gained in the mid-

An LDL/HDL Primer

There are several types of cholesterol, but in most cases, the American Heart Association concentrates on two—namely, HDL and LDL. LDL is known as the "bad" cholesterol because it builds up on artery walls and can lead to increased risk for cardiovascular disease and stroke. The American Heart Association considers a level of 130 mg/dL (milligrams per deciliter of blood) or less optimal for most people. HDL is the healthy cholesterol. It transports LDL cholesterol out of the bloodstream and deposits it in the liver, where it can be processed and excreted. High amounts of HDL (60 mg/dL or higher) give some protection from heart disease.

The ratio of HDL to total cholesterol is a very good way of measuring cardiovascular risk. Most physicians consider a ratio of 4 or under excellent. A person with total cholesterol of 200 mg/dL and an HDL of 50 mg/dL (total/HDL ratio = 4) has a lower risk of heart disease and stroke than someone with a total of 180 mg/dL and an HDL of 30 mg/dL (total/HDL ratio = 6).

section around menopause is new, but subcutaneous fat is still stored in the hips, thighs, or elsewhere.

V Is for Vicious

VISCERAL FAT GETS its name from the term *viscera*, which refers to the internal organs in the abdomen. It lies cloaked deep inside your body, where it wraps around your heart, liver, and other nearby major organs. Because it's sequestered beneath a layer of muscle, and it doesn't jiggle when you walk or always show up in your girth, some people call it "hidden fat." In fact, it's possible to be relatively thin and still have too much visceral fat. But this kind of fat can do far more than add inches to your waist: It can subtract years from your life. Carrying excess visceral fat is one of a complex group of symptoms collectively called metabolic syndrome, or syndrome X. The other symptoms are high cholesterol, high blood pressure, and elevated insulin levels. Having just one of these conditions contributes to your risk of serious disease, but your risk grows exponentially as the number of symptoms grows.

Visceral fat has been linked to a long list of adverse health conditions, the most serious of which are:

 High blood pressure, stroke, and heart disease
 Diabetes
 Breast cancer
 Dementia

One of the main reasons visceral fat is so deadly is its role in inflammation, a natural immune response that has lately been tied to almost every chronic disease you've ever heard of. Visceral fat secretes precursors to an inflammatory chemical that helps fuel the systemic process that exacerbates early symptoms of disease.

In fact, according to a study published in *Circulation: Journal of the American Heart Association*,[2] visceral fat may have a greater impact on the cardiovascular health of older women than overall obesity. Danish researchers found that women with excessive belly fat had a greater risk of atherosclerosis than those whose fat was stored mostly in their hips, thighs, and buttocks. Here's why.

▨ The proximity of visceral fat to your liver boosts production of LDL cholesterol—remember, the "lousy" kind—which collects in your arteries and forms plaque, a waxy substance.

▨ Over time, this waxy plaque becomes inflamed, causing swelling that narrows the arteries, restricting the passage of blood.

▨ The narrowing passageways increase blood pressure, straining your heart and potentially damaging tiny capillaries.

▨ The inflammation further increases your risk of blood clots, which can break loose and cause stroke.

But it gets worse. Visceral fat also contributes to insulin resistance, an early precursor to diabetes. Insulin resistance is a condition in which cells do not

How Fat Cells Work

A fat cell is like a tiny, expandable capsule—so tiny, it can't hold but a microscopic drop of fat. But fat cells prefer not to live alone; they cluster together like little gangs to become fatty tissue. They generally just chill out until they're called into action by precise biochemical signals, usually hormones and enzymes. When hormones and enzymes signal fat cells, they become active, releasing fat into the bloodstream to be used for different purposes.

When you overeat, those extra calories will travel right back into those deflated fat cells and fill them back up. No matter how much weight you lose or how many hours you spend in Spinning class, your fat cells will never disappear. A deflated balloon is still a balloon.

respond to insulin and the pancreas is forced to increase production to clear the bloodstream of glucose. Over time, insulin resistance can lead to full-blown diabetes, which can severely compromise the entire circulatory system and cause long-term issues with vision, memory, and wound healing.

As if that weren't enough, a Kaiser Permanente study comparing people with different levels of abdominal fat showed that those who had the *most* abdominal fat were 145 percent more likely to develop dementia, compared with people with the least amount of abdominal fat.[4] Why? Inflammation again, suggest researchers.

The One Number You Need to Remember

THE NATIONAL INSTITUTES OF HEALTH (NIH) have stated that a waist measurement of above 35 inches for women and 40 inches for men—*no matter how much you actually weigh*—is an unhealthy sign of excess visceral fat.[5]

A measurement that specifically reflects the concentration of fat around your belly is the waist-to-hip ratio, as opposed to measuring around your hips or thighs. In other words, it's just slightly more targeted to belly fat. Analyzing data from 27,000 people in 52 countries, scientists found that heart attack sufferers had BMIs similar to, but waist-to-hip ratios higher than, those who'd never had a heart attack. Which number would you rather track?

The waist-to-hip ratio compares the measurement of the narrowest part of your waist to the broadest section of your hips. Your waist measurement should be taken in the spot that falls between the rib cage and the hip bone, as viewed from the front.

Your hip measurement is truest if you turn sideways to the mirror and make sure you incorporate your derriere in the measurement. Now divide your waist measurement by your hip measurement. For example, a woman with a 30-inch waist and 37-inch hips has a waist/hip ratio of 0.81.

According to the Centers for Disease Control and Prevention, a healthy waist-to-hip ratio for women should not exceed 0.8.[6]

Other Ways to Measure Visceral Fat

PEOPLE CAN HAVE high amounts of visceral fat despite being at a normal weight because most of that fat is stored around the abdominal organs. This understanding is relatively new and describes those who are thin on the outside but have excess fat on the inside. It's hard to imagine that one could be thin and fat at the same time, but Jimmy Bell, PhD, a professor of molecular imaging at

The Benefits of Fat

From 2 to 5 percent of a man's body weight comes from essential fat, whereas for women, it's 10 to 13 percent. Fat is essential in humans for:

- Energy
- Maintaining proper hormone levels
- Regulating body temperature
- Protecting vital organs
- Fertility
- Bone growth

Body fat only becomes a problem when there's too much of it. At that point, it puts a strain on your heart and other organs and starts to interfere with your body confidence.

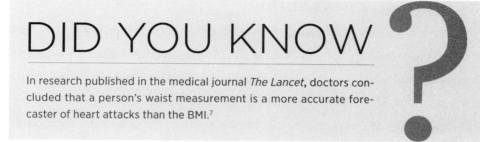

Imperial College, London, has shown that it is possible.[8] Dr. Bell and his team have been using magnetic resonance imaging (MRI) machines to scan nearly 800 people in an effort to produce what they call "fat maps." His findings will surprise you: About 45 percent of the thin women and 65 percent of the slim men he tested carried excess visceral fat.

As we understand more about the dangers of visceral fat, researchers are developing increasingly more accurate—and expensive—ways to measure it. The latest test, as we go to press with this book, is one that detects levels of a protein called RBP4 (retinol binding protein 4), which is produced in higher quantities in visceral fat, compared with subcutaneous fat. In overweight people, blood levels of RBP4 are double or triple the amount found in normal-weight people. But other tests are also used, including:

BIOELECTRICAL IMPEDANCE ANALYSIS

BIOELECTRICAL IMPEDANCE ANALYSIS (BIA) is portable, easy to use, and low-cost, compared with other procedures. A BIA involves circulating a very faint electrical current through the body. A device then calculates the resistance the current encounters as it travels through the body, computing body fat percentage based on height, weight, and speed of the current. A faster current translates to a lower body fat percentage because electricity travels faster through muscle (a greater percentage of water is found in muscle) than it does through fat.

SONOGRAM/ULTRASOUND

ULTRASOUND MACHINES SEND out high-frequency sound waves that reflect off body structures of different densities to create a picture called a sonogram. There is no radiation exposure with this test. A clear, water-based conducting gel is applied to the skin over the area being examined to improve the transmission of the sound waves. The ultrasound transducer (a handheld probe) is then moved over the abdomen to produce an image of what's inside.

DEXA

DUAL-ENERGY X-RAY ABSORPTIOMETRY (DEXA) uses less radiation than a CT scan to assess visceral fat and is less expensive. It's typically used to assess bone mineral density but can also be a valuable tool in assessing body composition.

MRI

MAGNETIC RESONANCE IMAGING (MRI) uses powerful magnets and radio waves to create pictures without the use of radiation. Images generated by MRI are generally superior to—but also generally more expensive than—computed tomagraphy (see next page) because they are more finely detailed.

DID YOU KNOW?

A recent Mayo Clinic study found that even a modest gain in visceral fat causes dysfunction of blood vessel linings. Even more surprising: The study participants were all lean and healthy. So you don't have to be "fat" to have an enemy in visceral fat.[9]

CT (CAT) Scan

A COMPUTED TOMOGRAPHY (CT) scanner uses radiation to create cross-sectional pictures of the body. The image results in a cross section of your belly that shows very clearly how much fat surrounds your organs. The latest scanners can image a whole body in less than 30 seconds.

Beyond Your Belly

REMEMBER, BY USING an inexpensive tape measure, you can most easily determine if your belly is endangering your health. But even if your belly measurement doesn't indicate a health risk, other things may motivate you to lose weight. Any reason is valid. No matter how or why your belly fat developed, you are clearly eager to get rid of it—and to keep it off! I'm going to offer you one of the best reasons—besides protecting your health—for trying this plan: the food! In the next chapter, you'll learn about the secret ingredients that make the *Flat Belly Diet* effective and delicious. These secret ingredients are called MUFAs.

READ A FLAT BELLY
SUCCESS
STORY

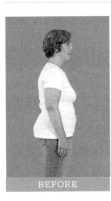

BEFORE

Donna Christiano

AGE: 47

POUNDS LOST:

7

IN 32 DAYS

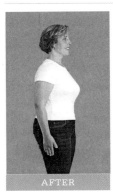

AFTER

ALL-OVER
INCHES LOST:

6.5

IT'S PRETTY AMAZING, WHEN YOU THINK ABOUT IT," EXCLAIMS Donna Christiano. "Seven pounds plus 6½ inches in a month—and never a day when I was hungry!" Donna calls the *Flat Belly Diet* the first weight-loss regimen she's followed that kept her satisfied 100 percent of the time. And she gives the MUFAs all the credit. "There's really something to them," she says. "I went away on vacation and stayed pretty true to the meal plan, but I couldn't always include a MUFA. And when I didn't, I found I was much hungrier than I thought I'd be."

But there's more, she adds. Since she started on this plan, she's become increasingly interested in doing what is good for her. In particular, she's much more conscious of eating healthy foods. She ate healthy food before but supplemented it with a lot of junk. On one of her earlier diets, she explains, foods were assigned a certain number of points, and she'd "spend" 15 on junk and 7 on what was good for her.

Not anymore. "I'm 47," she says. "I'm not getting any younger. This is the age when things start creeping up on you. So, for example, I used to love milk chocolate. Now I've started eating only dark chocolate. I try to optimize what I'm eating, too. Before, I put powdered creamer in my coffee, but now I realize that it's full of chemicals, so I've started using sweetened soy milk. I put cinnamon in coffee because it's another antioxidant. I add blueberries to my yogurt in an effort to get the biggest bang for the buck."

The best part, though, is that her belly is getting flatter. She relates a single anecdote to illustrate her success: She attended an exercise class with her neighbor Roseanne, whom she describes as tiny, tiny, and *tiny.* "She has a tiny waist, tiny hips. Just gorgeous. So we were in this class together, following along with the instructor, and I happened to glance in the mirror. I saw this woman with a really flat belly and I thought, 'Oh, that's Roseanne behind me.' Then I looked again. And I said to myself, 'Wait a minute! That person's wearing a red shirt. *I'm* wearing a red shirt. I think that's me!'" And it *was.*

"This diet just works for me," she raves. "Everything about it. I'm a snacker, and I like to eat every 4 hours. That's part of the diet. I love peanut butter for breakfast, and I can have 2 tablespoons. Two tablespoons! It's practically *sliding* off the bread and I think, 'Wow! This is so much food!' And the Snack Pack? Come *on*! Chocolate chips with 6 ounces of light yogurt and a piece of fruit? Chocolate chips *on a diet.* Can you imagine?"

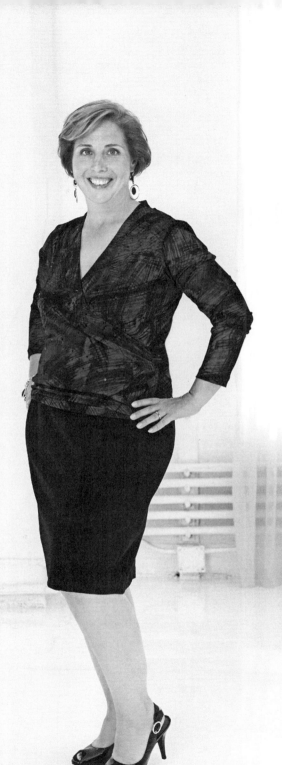

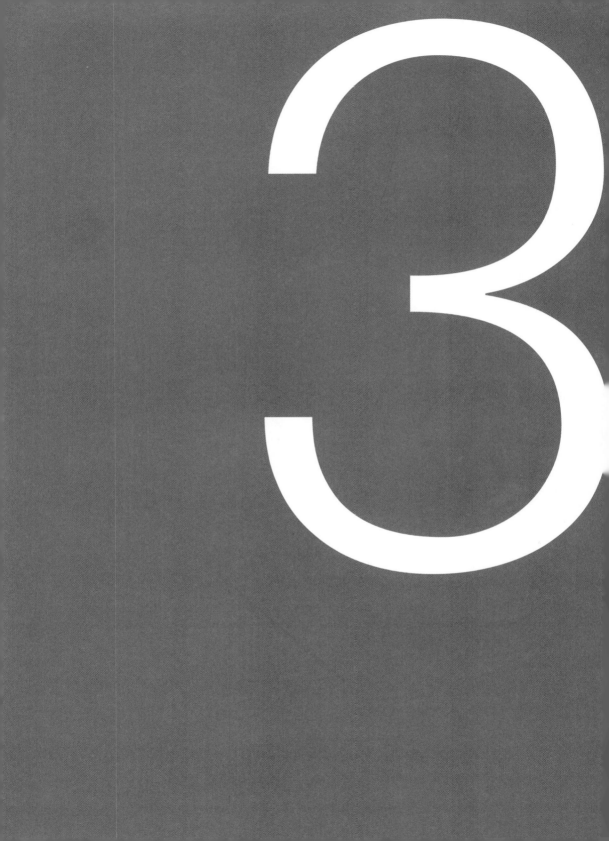

THE MAGIC OF
MUFAS

BELLY FAT MAY BE one of the most dangerous types of fat in the body, but I'm here to tell you that you don't have to live with it. You don't need to spend another day agonizing over your waistline and worrying about your rising disease risk, because there is an antidote to belly fat: MUFAs, otherwise known as monounsaturated fatty acids. There are five categories of MUFAs.

1. OILS
2. OLIVES
3. NUTS AND SEEDS
4. AVOCADOS
5. DARK CHOCOLATE

These miraculous foods hold the power to transform your body and your life. How? It's all in the name.

"MUFA" stands for **m**ono**u**nsaturated **f**atty **a**cid—a mouthful, I know—but to nutritionists like Cynthia, that mumbo jumbo perfectly describes why these plant-based fats are so healthful. Fatty acids are essentially the building blocks of all dietary fats, and like all organic elements, they're composed of atoms of carbon, oxygen, and hydrogen, all lined up in a particular way to form a chain. The term *saturated* is used when every one of the carbon atoms in the chain is bound to a hydrogen atom. This makes them solid or waxy at room temperature; in your body, they're sticky and inflexible. An *unsaturated* fat is one that isn't so tightly constructed and is therefore more flexible—this flexibility is the reason that unsaturated fats are "good" and saturated fats are "bad."

Think of saturated fats as sticks and unsaturated fats as strings. As saturated fats travel through your arteries, they bump and grind their way through, often getting stuck along the way. A recent study published in the *Journal of the American College of Cardiology* found that eating a meal high in saturated fat actually reduced the ability of blood vessels to expand and impaired blood flow.[1] This effect occurred just 3 hours after eating. Likewise, numerous studies have linked a long-term high intake of saturated fat to an increased risk of atherosclerosis (hardening of the arteries), heart disease, stroke, and other chronic diseases.

Since MUFAs are *un*saturated (i.e., more flexible), they can easily glide through your bloodstream without gumming up the works. This flexibility is just one reason why MUFAs are so healthful; a growing body of research indicates they may actually help to unclog and protect arteries from buildup.

MUFAs Make It Big

To REALLY UNDERSTAND how MUFAs rose to nutritional stardom and why "a MUFA at every meal" is such an important part of the *Flat Belly Diet,* I have to take you on a brief journey of the history of MUFAs (if you've been to Disney World, think Hall of Presidents, only about fats!). Once upon a time, in the not so distant past, all fats were sort of lumped together as being bad or fattening.

Recommendations from health professionals and the government based on the relationship between fats and heart disease were first introduced in the 1950s.[2] Ever since then, the emphasis has been on lowering saturated fat specifically, and the overall message has been to reduce total fat intake. One of the main tenets of the 1980 Dietary Guidelines was "Avoid too much fat, saturated fat, and cholesterol."[3] These government guidelines are revised every 5 years, but that wording remained in the next three versions. A full 15 years later, the 1995 report still stated, "Fat, whether from plant or animal sources, contains more than twice the number of calories of an equal amount of carbohydrate or protein. Choose a diet that provides no more than 30 percent of total calories from fat."[4]

This emphasis on total fat and the "less than 30 percent" wording left many people thinking "the less the better," creating scores of fat-phobic consumers who shunned not only butter and well-marbled meats but also vegetable oils, nuts, and peanut butter. This was a constant source of frustration for Cynthia, who knew about the dangers of cutting fat too low and had studied the health benefits of plant-based oils.

The 2000 Dietary Guidelines were slightly less restrictive. They stated, "Choose a diet that is low in saturated fat and cholesterol and *moderate* in total fat" and mentioned the healthfulness of plant-based fats, including oils and nuts.[5] But the message "Aim for a total fat intake of no more than 30 percent of calories" remained. It wasn't until a few years ago, in the 2005 Dietary Guidelines, that a minimum fat recommendation finally appeared.[6] The wording about fat in this version of the guidelines states, "Keep total fat intake between 20 to 35 percent of calories, with most fats coming from sources of polyunsaturated and monounsaturated fatty acids." Cynthia practically did cartwheels when she read it, particularly because she knew there was exciting research supporting the idea that not all fats were created equal.

The "Eat Less Fat" Backlash

STUDIES FROM THE 1950s to 1970s had indicated that a high total fat intake was associated with a greater risk of cardiovascular disease (CVD). According to the American Heart Association, CVD has been the number one killer in the United States every year for more than a century, except during the 1918 flu

Good Fats versus Bad Fats

Dietary fat is an important energy source. Used in the production of cell membranes and certain hormones, it's critical to the regulation of blood pressure, heart rate, blood vessel constriction, blood clotting, and the nervous system. Dietary fat aids the body in absorbing vitamins such as A, D, E, and K. But not all fats are created equal. Eating large amounts of the wrong fat is very hazardous to your health. But telling good fats from bad fats isn't so easy, unless you know what to look for:

THE HEALTHY

■ MONOUNSATURATED FAT (MUFA) remains liquid at room temperature but may start to solidify in the refrigerator.

■ POLYUNSATURATED FAT remains in liquid form both at room temperature and in the refrigerator. Foods high in polyunsaturated fats include vegetable oils, such as safflower, corn, sunflower, soy, and cottonseed oils.

■ OMEGA-3 FATTY ACIDS are an exceptionally healthy type of polyunsaturated fat found mostly in fat-rich seafoods such as salmon, mackerel, and herring. If you'd rather do your taxes than eat two fish meals a week (the recommended intake of healthy seafood), walnuts, flaxseeds, flaxseed oil, and, to a lesser degree, canola oil also contain omega-3 fatty acids.

pandemic.[7] And population data showed that Americans were consuming over a third of their total calories from fat. The 1971 National Health and Nutrition Examination Survey (NHANES) found that American women consumed about 36.9 percent of total calories from fat; and men, 36.1 percent.[8]

The message to reduce fat intake worked—sort of. By 2000, that percentage dropped to 32.8 percent for both sexes. Trouble is, total fat consumption in grams actually increased! The percentage shrank because total calorie intake rose—from roughly 1,542 calories to 1,877 for women and from about 2,450 calories to 2,618 for men. Most of those extra calories came from carbohydrates, causing the percentage of fat in the diet to shrink. According to the data, carbohydrate intake in grams jumped by a whopping 62 per day among women and 68 among men, while total fat grams increased among women by 6.5 grams and decreased among men by 5.3 grams. You probably remember news reports of fat-free, high-carbohydrate cookies, candies, and frozen yogurt flying off shelves;

THE UNHEALTHY

■ SATURATED FATS become solid or semi-solid at room temperature. The marbling in red meat is one example, as is a stick of butter. Saturated fat is found mostly in animal foods, but three vegetable sources are also high in saturated fat: coconut oil, palm (or palm kernel) oil, and cocoa butter. Keep in mind that it's almost impossible to get your saturated fat intake down to zero. Even olive oil contains 2 grams of saturated fat per tablespoon.

■ TRANS FATS raise LDL cholesterol and lower HDL cholesterol, increasing the risk of heart disease. They're quite possibly the most hated fats in all of fat-dom. Created when manufacturers hydrogenate liquid oils to increase their shelf life, they're found mostly in packaged products and nearly every food that contains shortening. Although nutrition facts labels must state trans fat content, the number is misleading, as manufacturers can legally claim zero grams trans fats even if up to $\frac{1}{2}$ gram per serving is present. Instead, look for the words "hydrogenated" or "partially hydrogenated" on ingredients lists to locate—and avoid—these deadly fats.

it was almost impossible to go food shopping without buying some sort of fat-free product. With all the emphasis on fat, most people saw a green light to eat high quantities of fat-free foods (like entire boxes of cookies, bags of jelly beans, or whole pints of fat-free frozen yogurt). And yes, obesity rates began to sky-rocket, rising from 14.5 percent in 1971 to 30.9 percent in 2000.

"Good" Fats to the Rescue

CLEARLY, THE "EAT LESS FAT" message wasn't the answer, and in the 1990s, scientists started to pay attention to the theory that eating moderate amounts of some types of fats could actually be protective, an idea first proposed by a University of Minnesota scientist named Ancel Keys, PhD, in his report called the Seven Countries Study.[9]

Between 1958 and 1970, Keys followed populations of men ages 40 to 59 in 18 areas of seven countries (United States, Japan, Italy, Greece, the Nether-lands, Finland, and Yugoslavia). His study looked at the men's diets, disease risk factors (such as blood cholesterol levels and blood pressure), and disease rates. It was the first to look at the links between diets and disease outcomes in different populations. The study was so important because it demonstrated the degree to which the composition of the diet could predict rates of coronary heart disease. The major conclusion was that—hello!—a high fat intake was *not* associated with higher rates of heart disease.

The standout area was Crete, the largest of the Greek islands. Cretan men had the lowest rates of heart disease of all populations observed in the Seven Countries Study, as well as the highest average life span, despite consuming 37 percent of their calories from fat (Finland and the United States had the highest number of deaths from heart disease). Throughout the study, Keys observed that the Cretans' diets were consistent. They consumed the same types of traditional Greek meals they had been enjoying for centuries, including lots of fruits, vegetables (especially greens), nuts, beans, fish, moderate amounts of wine and cheese, small quantities of grass-fed meat, milk, eggs, some whole grains, and plenty of MUFA-rich olive oil and olives. Cretan people consume on average 25 liters (100 cups) of olive oil per person each year.

Viva la Olive Oil!

THE FASCINATING FINDINGS in Crete put olive oil at center stage, and finally, the idea that some fats are healthful began to gain acceptance. Dozens of Mediterranean diet studies focusing on olive oil followed, with amazing conclusions. A Greek study concluded that the exclusive use of olive oil was associated with a 47 percent lower likelihood of having cardiovascular disease, even after adjustments were made to account for BMI, smoking, physical activity level, educational status, a family history of heart disease, high blood pressure, high cholesterol, and diabetes.[10] Another published in the *American Journal of Clinical Nutrition* in the late 1990s looked at the effects of long-term olive oil intake and blood triglyceride levels on a group of healthy men.[11] The olive oil group had significantly reduced levels of LDL cholesterol.

Numerous controlled studies have found that olive oil can lower circulating LDL levels, or prevent cholesterol from hardening. That's critical, because hardening is the beginning of the domino effect that results in artery damage and disease. But as more and more studies were conducted, it became clear that while olive oil is amazingly healthful, a great deal of its protective power lies in its MUFAs, which are also found in other plant fats, including nuts and avocado.

Eventually, research began to shift from olive oil to MUFAs and led to findings that MUFA protection extends far beyond cholesterol and heart disease. MUFAs have now been linked to reduced rates of type 2 diabetes, metabolic syndrome, breast cancer, and inflammation, plus healthier blood pressure, brain function, lung function, body weight, and—you guessed it—belly fat. In fact, when Cynthia showed me the stack of published studies on MUFAs specifically, I could hardly believe my eyes—it was at least as thick as this entire book. So in the interest of not overwhelming you (and saving a few trees), I've included a few of the most compelling studies. I think this summary will help you see why we're so over the moon about MUFAs.

MUFAs Protect Your Heart

▨ French scientists tested the effects of replacing some dietary carbohydrates with MUFAs without reducing calories. They found that the MUFA-rich diet produced better effects on blood triglyceride levels and other markers for cardiovascular disease.[12]

▨ Johns Hopkins researchers compared the effects of three healthful diets, each with reduced saturated fat intake, on blood pressure and blood fat levels over 6 weeks, without allowing for weight loss.[13] The first diet was rich in carbohydrates, the second high in protein (with about half from plant sources), and the third high in MUFAS. They found that the protein and MUFA diets further lowered blood pressure, improved blood fat levels, and reduced the estimated risk of CVD.

▨ Pennsylvania State University faculty compared the CVD risk profile of an average American diet to four different cholesterol-lowering diets: an American Heart Association/National Cholesterol Education Program Step II diet and three high-MUFA diets.[14] The Step II diet and all of the high-MUFA diets lowered total cholesterol by 10 percent and LDL cholesterol by 14 percent. The MUFA diets also lowered triglyceride concentrations by 13 percent (while the step II increased them by 11 percent) and did not lower "good" HDL cholesterol (the Step II diet lowered HDL by 4 percent).

University of Barcelona scientists compared the short-term effects of two Mediterranean diets versus a low-fat diet on markers of cardiovascular risk.[15] Compared with the low-fat diet, the mean changes in blood sugar, blood pressure, and cholesterol were significantly better in both the MUFA-rich olive oil–based Mediterranean diet and the MUFA-rich, nut-based Mediterranean groups.

The research on MUFAs and heart health is so compelling that a daily MUFA target has now become part of the standard scientific protocol for preventing and managing CVD risk. The Therapeutic Lifestyle Changes (TLC) plan, developed by the National Heart, Lung, and Blood Institute (a branch of the National Institutes of Health), is designed to reduce the risk of coronary heart disease.[16] It recommends a total fat intake of 25 to 35 percent of daily calories, with saturated fat at no more than 7 percent of calories and MUFA up to 20 percent of total calories.

MUFAs Ward Off Type 2 Diabetes

Spanish researchers studied the effects of three weight-maintenance diets on carbohydrate and fat metabolism and insulin levels in overweight subjects by randomly assigning them to 28-day diets high in either saturated fat, monounsaturated fat (MUFAs), or carbohydrate.[17] Fasting blood sugar levels fell on both the MUFA-rich and carb-rich diets, but the MUFA diet also improved insulin sensitivity and boosted HDL cholesterol levels.

At Indiana University, scientists treated type 2 diabetes patients with either a MUFA-rich weight-reducing diet and or a low-fat, high-carbohydrate weight-loss diet for a 6-week period.[18] Both groups lost pounds, but the MUFA group had a greater decrease in total cholesterol and triglyceride levels and a smaller drop in HDL cholesterol—and those results were sustained even after the group was allowed to regain the weight.

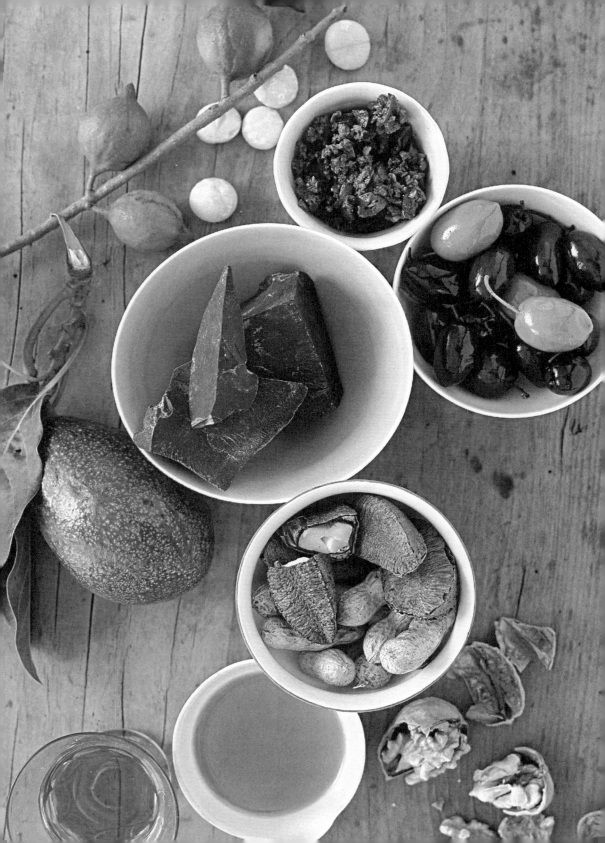

CHOOSE YOUR MUFA

These marvelous monounsaturated fat–packed foods can help you live a long, healthy life with less belly fat. But these foods also provide a host of other beneficial nutrients.

1. Oils: The health benefits of the *Flat Belly Diet*–recommended oils (canola, safflower, sesame, soybean, walnut, flaxseed, sunflower, olive, and peanut) differ depending on the nut, seed, or fruit they were pressed from. Flaxseed and walnut oil are both rich sources of alpha-linolenic acid, which your body converts into omega-3 fatty acids. Extra virgin olive oil has strong antibacterial properties and can even kill *H. pylori,* the bacterium that causes most peptic ulcers and some types of stomach cancer.[19] In addition, olive oil contains phytochemicals called polyphenols, which also help prevent cardiovascular disease and cancer and reduce inflammation in the body. Canola, sesame, sunflower, safflower, and soybean oils are all rich in vitamin E.

2. Olives: In addition to their MUFAs, olives are a good source of iron, vitamin E, copper (a mineral that protects your nerves, thyroid, and connective tissue), and fiber (to regulate your digestive system, help control blood sugar levels, and manage blood cholesterol).

3. Nuts and Seeds: Like oils, the health benefits of the Flat Belly nuts and seeds are numerous and varied. Sunflower seeds are a good source of linoleic acid. In a recent study, women who had the highest intakes of linoleic acid had a 23 percent lower risk of heart disease, compared with those with the lowest intakes.[20] The omega-3 fatty acids in walnuts have been linked to protection against inflammation, heart disease, asthma, and arthritis and improved cognitive function. And pistachios have been shown to help keep blood pressure down in stressful situations. Overall, nuts and seeds are good sources of many key nutrients, including protein, fiber, iron, zinc, magnesium, copper, B vitamins, and vitamin E.

4. Avocados: Avocados are packed with lutein, which may help maintain healthy eyes, as well as beta-sitosterol, a natural plant sterol that may help keep cholesterol down. Adding avocado to salads and salsas has been shown to more than double the absorption of carotenoids, antioxidants linked to lower risk of heart disease and macular degeneration, a leading cause of blindness.[21] Avocados are also rich in fiber, vitamin K (which helps clot blood), potassium (which regulate blood pressure), and heart-protective folate.

5. Dark Chocolate: Dark chocolate is rich in flavanols and proanthocyanins, both of which boost good HDL cholesterol levels. It also contains natural substances that help control insulin levels and relax blood vessels, lowering blood pressure, and provides important minerals including copper, magnesium, potassium, calcium, and iron.

MUFAs Cut Metabolic Syndrome Risk

Researchers from the department of medicine at Columbia University in New York studied 52 men and 33 women with metabolic syndrome (defined as any combination of low HDL cholesterol, high triglycerides, or high insulin).[22] Over 7 weeks they were randomly assigned to either a typical American diet with 36 percent of calories from fat or two additional diets, in which 7 percent of the calories from saturated fat were replaced with either carbohydrate or MUFAs. They found that LDL cholesterol was reduced with both the lower-saturated-fat diets, but MUFAs protected the HDL and lowered triglycerides, which were significantly higher with the high-carbohydrate diet.

MUFAs Reduce Inflammation

IN A NUTSHELL, inflammation is our immune system's response to stress, injury, or illness. It's a known trigger for premature aging and disease, but MUFAs are effective at quelling its "flames."

A Spanish study focused on a large group of men and women at high risk for CVD.[23] It found that the consumption of particular Mediterranean foods, including MUFA-rich virgin olive oil and nuts, was associated with lower blood concentrations of inflammatory markers.

In an Italian study, the effect of a Mediterranean-style diet on inflammatory markers in patients with metabolic syndrome was studied.[24] Over 3 years, researchers randomly assigned nearly 200 men and women with metabolic syndrome to either a Mediterranean-style diet rich in whole grains, fruits, vegetables, and MUFA-rich nuts and olive oil, or a "prudent" diet composed of 50 to 60 percent carbohydrate, 15 to 20 percent protein, and 30 percent or less fat (the old Dietary Guidelines standard). After 2 years, patients following the Mediterranean-style diet, who had consumed more total grams of MUFA and fiber per day, had a greater decrease in mean body weight. The high-MUFA diet also significantly reduced blood concentrations of inflammatory markers and decreased insulin resistance.

MUFAs Lower Your Risk of Breast Cancer

In a study published in the journal *Archives of Internal Medicine,* scientists from the department of medical epidemiology at the Karolinska Institute in Stockholm, Sweden, looked at data on 61,471 women ages 40 to 76 years from two counties in central Sweden who did not have any previous diagnosis of breast cancer.[25] After following the women over time and evaluating both their diets and incidence of breast cancer, they found an inverse association between MUFAs and breast cancer risk. There was a 45 percent reduction in the risk of developing breast cancer for each 10-gram increment of MUFA consumed daily.

MUFAs Keep Your Brain Healthy

Scientists in the department of geriatrics in the Center for Aging Brain at the University of Bari in Italy set out to study the relationships between diet and age-related changes in cognitive functions. The researchers looked at a sample of 5,632 people between the ages of 65 and 84 in eight regions of Italy.[26] They used a battery of standardized tests to assess cognitive functions, selective attention, and memory and evaluated the subjects' diets and found that those with the highest percentage of calories from MUFAs had the greatest protection against cognitive decline.

Another Italian study, led by scientists at the center's Memory Unit, investigated the role of diet in age-related cognitive decline (ARCD) by studying an elderly population in southern Italy that consumed a typical Mediterranean diet.[27] They also concluded that high intake of MUFAs warded off ARCD.

MUFAs Extend Your Life

■ Several studies have looked at the link between MUFA intake and life expectancy. An $8\frac{1}{2}$-year follow-up to the Italian Longitudinal Study on Aging investigated the possible role of MUFAs and other foods in protecting against all-causes mortality.[28] Among subjects without dementia between the ages of 65 and 84, scientists found that a higher MUFA intake was associated with an increase of survival, and there was no effect found in any other selected food group.

MUFAs Target Belly Fat

■ A 2007 study published in the journal *Diabetes Care* found that a MUFA-rich diet prevented central body fat distribution, compared with a high-carbohydrate and high-saturated-fat diet of the same calorie level.[29]

■ Australian researchers randomly assigned overweight men to various 4-week diets composed of the same calorie level with different amounts of saturated, monounsaturated, and polyunsaturated fat. The MUFA-rich diet resulted in lower total body weight and body fat. The authors concluded that a

SASS FROM SASS

"Try My Favorite MUFA."

I keep a selection of MUFAs in my office at all times, but there's one stash I never let get too low: dry-roasted pumpkin seeds, my favorites. I love to eat them one at a time. It's amazing how long it can take to eat 2 tablespoons when you eat them one after another versus downing a handful at once. When I crack them between my teeth, I can sometimes feel the oil ooze out a little—that's because pumpkin seeds aren't as "meaty" as, say, almonds, so the oil is less dispersed throughout the seed. —*Cynthia*

high-MUFA diet can induce a significant loss of body weight and fat mass without a change in total calorie or fat intake.

■ Another Aussie study compared postmeal body fat burning rates after two breakfasts: one with saturated fat from cream and one with MUFA from olive oil.[30] The MUFA group had a significantly higher fat-burning rate in the 5 hours following the MUFA breakfast, particularly in the subjects with greater abdominal fat.

The Other Antidote to Belly Fat: Attitude

OF COURSE, THE *Flat Belly Diet* isn't only about food. Before we get to the eating plan, I want you to understand the one factor that will be key to making your dream of a flat belly come true—and that's your state of mind. Your emotions, stress level, and body image all play a role in how and when you eat—and even how and where you put on weight. That's right—your emotional state can actually cause you to store belly fat. In the next chapter, we'll explore this mind-belly connection in depth and reveal the secret to succeeding on the Flat Belly Diet. But for now, let's bask in the glorious knowledge that flattening your belly may be as easy as drizzling olive oil on your next salad, spreading peanut butter on a cracker, or—oh, yes—licking melted chocolate off your fingertips.

READ A FLAT BELLY
SUCCESS
STORY

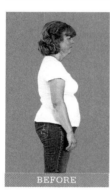

BEFORE

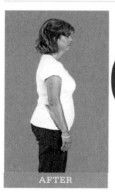

AFTER

Diane Kaspareck

AGE: 52

POUNDS LOST:

6.5
IN 32 DAYS

ALL-OVER INCHES LOST:

6.25

"FOR ME, LEARNING THAT PREVENTION HAD PUT OUT A call for participants in their new *Flat Belly Diet* turned out to be both timely and an unexpected blessing in so many ways," says Diane Kaspareck. The 52-year-old nurse, who also happens to be a cancer survivor, calls her cancer experience a defining time in her life. As she reached the fifth anniversary of her diagnosis, she decided, "It's time to shelve the *survivor* identity, and get on with my life."

Part of that decision included going on the *Flat Belly Diet*. "It was just at that time that I heard about the diet," she recalls, "so I decided to give myself a 5-year anniversary gift." Her goal was to shore up her health, shed her excess pounds, and return her body to a complete state of balance. "It was one of the first times in my life I had ever done anything that was *only* for me."

The first weekend on the diet, Diane sent her husband and son off to the beach, and she stayed at home alone to concentrate on the food plan. "I realized there is a learning curve with it, so I started very methodically, shopping for the food and making the meals and sitting down by myself to enjoy them. I decided to start walking every day, too, and it all just took off from there.

"It's interesting," she says. "As you start to deal with your health issues and get better at it, you start treating yourself better. You connect more to yourself in a lot of different ways. Even mentally you're feeling better. Things aren't as overwhelming, maybe because you have more energy."

She's in thrall of that newfound energy. In the past, she used to come home from work and plop onto the sofa at 4 p.m., just in time for *Oprah*. "That was it for me—I was done for the evening. I was tired and maybe even a little bit depressed." Things are different now. The food she's eating and the weight loss have energized her. She's out evenings and wanting to do more and more. "It's as if I have gotten back another 6 hours a day of my life," she says.

"I know it's just a diet, but I feel so good. And I'm so much happier. Cancer takes away some of your control, but now I feel as though I have a handle on a controllable issue. My body is in a really good equilibrium as far as nutrition, and I feel calmer and more relaxed—like nothing scary is going to jump out of the closet at me."

Diane lost only 6$\frac{1}{2}$ pounds on the first 32 days of the *Flat Belly Diet,* but her muscle mass and her body fat percentage changed. She feels losing slowly is a good thing. "Do I want to lose more? Sure," she says. "But I realized in the big picture, that's just how it is. You don't gain it or lose it overnight. I really feel as though I've got some fabulous new habits that will stay with me. And I'm going to keep going until I lose every pound I set out to lose."

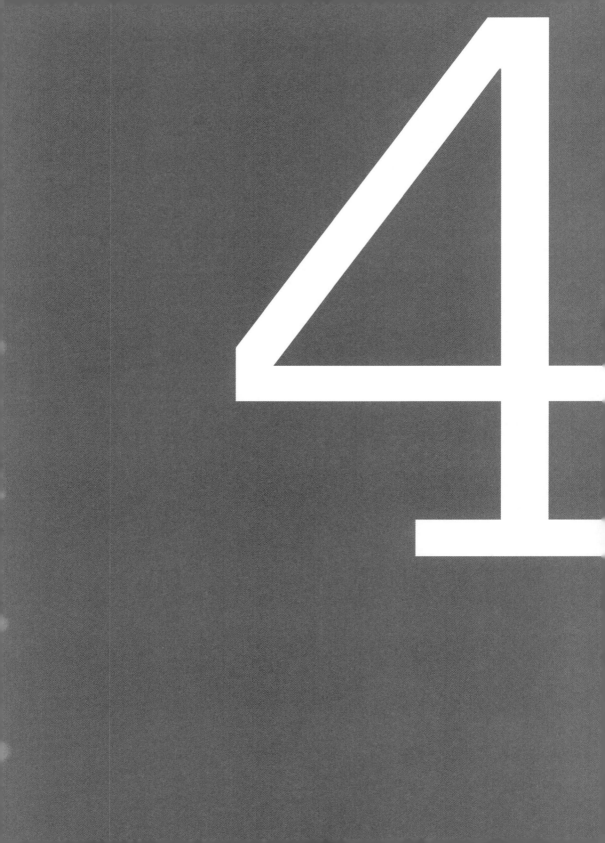

THE MIND-BELLY CONNECTION

THE RELATIONSHIP BETWEEN mind and body is pretty solid. Understanding how they work together is key to reaching your weight loss—or any—lifestyle goal. Why? Consider the role your emotions, attitudes, and feelings play in what you eat, how much you eat, and when you eat it.

I clearly recall the day it dawned on me that my relationship to food is profoundly affected by my body image. It was back in the 1980s, and it was all about a mirror. I had just moved into my first apartment and, needing to give myself the once-over and ensure that my skirt wasn't tucked into my pantyhose before heading out each day, I bought a full-length mirror and propped it against a wall.

For the next month, I smiled happily at the longer, leaner image I saw every morning. Wondering if I'd magically dropped 5 pounds on move-in day, I weighed myself on the scale at the gym. Nope, hadn't lost an ounce. But boy, did I feel thinner! I was so motivated by this state of affairs that over the next couple of weeks, I decided to maintain the healthy momentum. I ran farther, ate smaller portions, skipped desserts, and took fewer dips into the office candy bowl.

Then I finally got around to hanging the mirror properly. That's when I discovered that tilting a mirror against a wall (with the bottom of the glass closer to you than the top) makes your reflection appear longer and leaner. When I hung that sucker flush and turned to see my profile, I came face-to-face with reality. What I saw was hardly "fat"—just slightly less *flat*. Still, it was a major blow to my body confidence. I drove straight to McDonald's and ordered a Big Mac®. True story.

At *Prevention*, we know from years of experience talking to women who have tried many diets that attitude, emotions, thoughts, feelings, and practically everything mind-related all influence the foods you choose to eat and the way you eat them. That's why the *Flat Belly Diet* is about engaging your mind as much as your tastebuds. Only if your brain is on board will you enjoy success.

Conquer Emotional Eating

PHYSIOLOGICALLY SPEAKING, your appetite is controlled by biochemical signals that tell your brain that you're hungry and need to eat or satisfied and can stop. The problem is, we've all learned to override those signals. We eat not only when we're hungry but also when we're happy or sad, relaxed, or anxious.

To get a handle on emotional eating, you need to understand why you do it. For one thing, many of us have been conditioned to believe that food can bring comfort (remember getting a lollipop after a shot at the doctor's?). And it does, at least in the short term. As adults, many of us turn to food to relieve feelings of stress. Snacking is a common response to boredom, anxiety, anger, and, yes, loneliness. (I've been known to lean on spoonfuls of peanut butter when faced with writer's block.)

For many of us, years of eating to address everything *but* an empty stomach means we have to relearn what actual hunger feels like. Although we often don't recognize it, the line between emotional hunger and *true* hunger is actually quite clear. Researchers from the University of Texas Counseling and Mental Health Center have identified five ways to differentiate between the two:[1]

1. Emotional hunger comes on suddenly, while physical hunger is gradual.

2. Physical hunger is felt below the neck (growling stomach), while emotional hunger is felt above the neck (a craving for ice cream).

3. When only a certain food like pizza or chocolate will meet your need, your "hunger" is born of emotion. When your body requires fuel, you're more open to other food options.

4. Emotional hunger wants to be satisfied instantly. Physical hunger can wait.

5. Emotional hunger leaves guilt in its wake. Physical hunger doesn't.

Recognizing these signals can help you distinguish an emotional need for food from a physical one. The next time a craving strikes, try this: Tune out the signals coming from the neck up. Are you physically hungry? Ask yourself what you're feeling emotionally and how you can meet these mental (versus physical) needs.

The real cure for emotional eating is developing effective coping strategies, not just seeking out distractions. Here's an example: When you're sad and craving ice cream, cleaning out your closet may direct you away from the freezer, but it won't help you exorcise that melancholy feeling. Too often, we fail to take the very important steps of first identifying the emotions we're experiencing and, second, *feeling* them. If you're feeling sad, watch a tearjerker and allow yourself to have a good cry. Or call a close friend who's eager to hear you out in such times. Addressing the emotion rather than avoiding it is the best way to release yourself from the desire to eat.

Address the Stress Factor

WHEN SCIENTISTS STUDY STRESS, they always differentiate between two types: *acute,* or short-term, and *chronic,* or long-term. An example of *chronic* stress could be having a job you dislike but feel you can't escape from. An example of short-term, or *acute,* stress? It might be as ordinary as being late for a meeting or as life-threatening as almost being hit by a car.

Back in the Stone Age, our species' very survival depended on the ability to respond instantly to short-term stresses like being chased by predators. Today, we're still equipped with a hair-trigger mechanism that overrides our rational minds in an emergency or when we feel threatened. We call it the fight-or-flight response, and it's no different if the stressor is a ravenous beast or an impatient boss. Here's how it works.

THE BIOLOGY OF ACUTE STRESS

STRESS RESPONSES BEGIN in the nervous system. The central nervous system (CNS) responds to orders from the conscious mind, while the autonomic nervous system (ANS) functions independently. If you decide, for example, to take a picture of a friend with your cell phone, the CNS puts into play all the actions involved in completing the task, from having the idea to snapping the shutter. Meanwhile, you will continue to breathe (without having to think about it), and

DID YOU KNOW?

Researchers at the University of Minnesota, in a study of 1,800 dieting adults, found that those who weighed themselves every day lost an average of 12 pounds over 2 years, while those who only weighed themselves once per week lost an average of 6 pounds.[2]

your body will continue to go about the business of digesting food, pumping blood, and fending off harmful bacteria. Your ANS governs these functions, operating without a single conscious thought or action on your part.

Within the ANS, there are two branches: the sympathetic nervous system (SNS) and the parasympathetic nervous system (PNS). The first revs you up, and the second calms you down. Say, for example, you're crossing a busy intersection and see an out-of-control car heading straight for you. You don't consciously order your heart to pump faster and deliver more blood to your muscles so they can react with more force to get you out of the way; you just naturally jump onto the curb. In that mere millisecond, your brain perceives the threat and kicks the SNS into high gear. Here's what happens next.

■ The hypothalamus in the brain sends a message to your adrenal glands near your kidneys, which pump out the hormones adrenaline and cortisol (more on this later).

■ Adrenaline increases your heartbeat to twice its normal speed, sending extra blood to the brain, as well as to the major muscles in your arms and legs—so you're better able to dodge that moving car.

■ Your memory gets sharper.

■ Your immune system goes on alert—in case it's needed to fight infection from an impending wound.

- Your arteries narrow—so if you're injured, you'll lose less blood.
- Narrowed arteries cause an increase in blood pressure.
- Your pupils dilate and your vision becomes more acute.
- Your digestive system slows down.
- Insulin production ramps up, overriding signals from adrenaline to burn fat, and encourages the body to store it in anticipation of future needs.

All this happens to get you safely out of the way of that car barreling toward you—and, once upon a time, to enable our ancestors to dodge that hungry saber-toothed tiger intent on landing its next meal. When the immediate threat is over, so is the short-term stress. That's when the PNS steps in, releasing calming hormones, and your body returns once again to equilibrium.

THE HIGH PRICE OF CHRONIC STRESS

UNLIKE ACUTE STRESS, which has a beginning and an end, chronic stress is ongoing. When your marriage hits a rough patch, your child has trouble in school, you finally get that promotion and your workload doubles, your aging parents suddenly need a lot more care—or all of these things happen at once!—that is chronic stress. The problem is, your body still reacts as if these stresses were acute, yet—and here's the important distinction—there's no calming period. The SNS just keeps doing its stuff, keeping you in a state of heightened physiological arousal as if your very life were being threatened, 24/7. The more your body's stress response system is activated, the more difficult it is to switch off. And that's a major concern, given that anywhere from 60 to 90 percent of illness is stress-related. Here's how the stress/health connection works.

In times of stress, the adrenal glands secrete an abundance of cortisol. Normally, cortisol's role is to *regulate* blood pressure, cardiovascular function, and metabolism. Your body can easily handle the occasional burst of cortisol triggered by an acute or high-stress moment—no problem there. It's when the stress is chronic and a steady stream of cortisol begins to flow into your bloodstream that things start to go bad. Too much cortisol weakens your immune system, puts your heart into overdrive, and raises your blood pressure. A consistently high level of circulating stress hormones adversely affects brain function as well, especially memory. And excessive cortisol can also interfere with "feel-good" neurotransmitters such as dopamine and serotonin, making you more vulnerable to depression.

Cortisol and Belly Fat

REST ASSURED, I haven't forgotten why you're here. This is a book about belly fat, so let's turn our attention now to cortisol and its affinity for our bellies. Research has shown that cortisol not only stimulates the appetite but specifically induces cravings for sugar and fat—the most easily burned "fuels." This helps explain why many of us eat when we're stressed; it also sheds some light

Signs of Chronic Stress

- Headaches
- Frequent upset stomach, indigestion, gas pain, diarrhea, or appetite changes
- Feeling as though you might cry
- Muscular tension
- Tightness in your chest and a feeling that you can't catch your breath
- Feeling nervous or sad
- Feeling irritable and angry
- Having problems at work or in your normal relationships
- Sleep disturbance: either insomnia or hypersomnia (sleeping too much)
- Apathy (lack of interest, motivation, or energy)
- Mental or physical fatigue
- Frequent illness
- Hives or skin rashes
- Tooth grinding
- Feeling faint or dizzy
- Ringing in the ears
- Disruptions/skips in menstrual cycle; unusually severe PMS or menopausal symptoms

on why it's the pint of ice cream we reach for rather than a nice crisp apple.

But here's the kicker: Cortisol also signals the body to *store* fat centrally, around the organs. That's right—at your belly. It's nature's way of ensuring that resources are readily and easily available for fuel when the body needs them to perform life-preserving exertion or, for that matter, withstand famine. This all makes even more sense when you take into account the fact that abdominal fat has both a greater blood supply (so cortisol travels there quickly) and more receptors for cortisol.

You *Can* Take Control!

AFTER EACH OF my life's most terrifying moments—piano recital at 9, gymnastic meet at 12, first television appearance at 25—my mother always told me, to my great surprise, that I didn't look the least bit nervous. If she only knew what was happening inside! As I've gotten older, I have learned a few tried-and-true methods for managing the day-to-day pressures of running a magazine, raising my daughters, and tackling hundreds of other projects, like writing this book. My main tactic is to heap lots of gratitude onto the world's greatest husband and New Jersey's best nanny. After that, I shoot for regular exercise, laughing really hard at least once a day, and actually saying the words "I am so lucky to have you" to my husband, Steve, and daughters, Sophia and Olivia, whenever I can.

For me, these tactics give me focus, perspective, and calm (on most days of the week!). It's easy for me to tell you to reduce stress by "finding a hobby" or "asking your children to do the dishes more often," but how helpful are these suggestions, really? *Prevention*'s 2007 Picture of Health winner writes in her gratitude journal every day. My husband kayaks on the quietest lake he can find. And an editor friend meditates every morning—an idea I love but an activity I just can't wrap my brain around . . . yet. (I'm working on it.) My point is: Since your sources of stress are personal, so should be the ways you counteract their effects.

However, researchers have targeted certain behaviors that will be helpful for most women trying to manage busy lives, deflect anxiety, and find happiness. These seven stress-busting strategies will not only help you feel calm and live a more relaxing existence but will prevent stress-induced weight gain in the process. Use this list like a tool kit. The more tools you use, the more you'll benefit.

Get Calm! 7 Stress-Busting Strategies

1. GET MORE SLEEP. At the turn of the 20th century, the average American typically slept about 9 hours a night. Can you imagine? Nowadays most of us are lucky to get 7. This doesn't just make you tired; it can make you stressed—and fat. Consistently depriving yourself of rest subjects your body to a constant level of elevated stress. Sleep deprivation results in reduced levels of leptin, a

Not All Stress Is Harmful

Believe it or not, Some kinds of acute stress are beneficial. Ohio State University researchers found that stress from engaging in a memory task activated the immune system, whereas the stress created by passively watching a violent video weakened immunity (as measured by salivary concentration of sIgA, a major immune factor). These results suggest that minor mental challenges and deadlines at work could help strengthen your body's defenses.[5]

protein that regulates body fat and increases ghrelin, which stimulates appetite. So not getting enough sleep causes your body to store fat, slows your metabolism, and makes you want to eat more. Your body must have enough downtime to revitalize and replenish its reserves. This is especially true for anyone on a diet, because if you're in any way sleep deprived, it's that much more difficult to summon the physical energy and mental focus to stick to any diet *or* exercise plan. I urge you: If you do nothing else on this list, put getting a good night's sleep at the top of your *Flat Belly* to-do list.

■ Slip on some socks. The instant warmup provided by socks widens blood vessels and allows your body to transfer heat from its core to the extremities, cooling you slightly. This induces sleep, says Phyllis Zee, PhD, director of sleep disorders at Northwestern University's Feinberg School of Medicine. If you wear an old-fashioned nightcap, you can achieve the same result.[6]

■ Stay on schedule. People who follow regular daily routines report fewer sleep problems than those with more unpredictable lifestyles, according to a study from the University of Pittsburgh Medical Center. Recurring time cues will synchronize your body rhythms and sleep-wake cycles, explains Lawrence Epstein, MD.[7]

■ Go dark. Any light will signal the brain to wake up, but "blue light" from your cell phone and your clock's digital display is the worst offender. Dim your clock and eliminate lighted devices from the bedroom.

2. GET SOME DISTANCE. Take note of the things that cause you chronic stress—and, when possible, sidestep them. When emotions run high, you may find yourself biting your nails, leaning on your car horn, forgetting important appointments, even yelling at your kids. If you think about what's bothering you—really think about it—you'll most likely find it's not your nails or your children or the traffic that's the problem. It's that you've maxed out what I like to think of as your stress reserves, and you need to interrupt the stress cycle. When this happens, remove yourself from the scene. Just walk away. Literally. Go around the block or just into the next room. If even that is impossible, simply close your eyes, count to 10, and breathe deeply. Those few simple moments might give you a chance to process strong emotions before they overwhelm you. Physically, you should feel better almost immediately.

3. GET MOVING. EVERY DAY. Studies show that even 10 minutes of physical activity will help reduce levels of cortisol in the bloodstream. Exercise changes your body's biochemistry, triggering the brain to produce beta-endorphins, chemicals that calm you down, regulate your stress hormones, and make you feel good. So the next time you feel like pulling your hair out or reaching for a fistful of Fritos, head for the door and take a bike ride or even just a quick walk around the block. A little exercise may not solve the problem at hand, but it will certainly help you cope with it.

4. GET CONNECTED. Talking with others can defuse your feelings of tension, but studies have shown that even just being in someone's company—without saying a word—helps alleviate stress. It also promotes good health: Research shows that people who maintain personal and community connections have better health than those who don't.

An important caveat to keep in mind: Only spend time with people who leave

Walk for Deep Sleep

A little walking goes a long way toward getting a sound night's sleep. When researchers studied more than 700 men and women, they found that those who walked at least six blocks a day at a moderate pace were one-third less likely to have sleeping problems than those who walked shorter distances. Those who walked at a brisker pace were most likely of all to enjoy sound sleep. Other studies show that a regular walking program is as effective at improving sleep as medication. For walking workouts and a full calendar, go to prevention.com/walking.[8]

you energized, not emotionally drained. If there is any doubt about which is which, ask yourself this question after you've been with the person: Did I have fun, or did I work hard to make sure my *friend* had fun? Of course, the answer to both of these questions can be yes, but if the answer to the first question is no, that's a pretty good clue that you need to find someone else to spend time with. Emotionally draining people—or, in the popular terminology of today, toxic people—do very little to boost your self-confidence or keep you on track toward your goals.

5. GET POSITIVE. Lose the negative self-talk. I'm referring to that little voice in your head that passes judgment on your every move. Whenever you catch yourself thinking, "I'll never get this report done" or "My house is a filthy wreck," stop yourself and redirect your thinking. Instead, replay the thought but with a positive spin: "I will do my absolute best to meet this deadline" and "I love this house for all its wonderful memories." Forcing these thoughts might feel silly, but I promise you: It will help you feel more in control of your life, and it will build your self-respect and self-confidence. And, as we now know, that is integral to achieving your health and weight-loss goals!

Stop the Time Suck

A little time management can go a long way to remedy stress. Keep in mind: Time management isn't necessarily about doing more—it's about doing more of the things you *want* to do. Try keeping a time tracker for a day or two to find out where your time is really going.

Set up a daily timetable on your computer or in a journal, broken into 15-minute blocks. Track what you do in each block of time from when you wake up to when you go to bed, and evaluate each day. Seeing how you actually spend your time throughout the day may help you determine how you can make small changes that reduce your stress and improve your ability to fit in healthy meals, more physical activity, or just a little downtime.

SASS FROM SASS

"The Mental Tweak That Will Set You Up for Success"

If there's one thing I've learned from my years of nutrition counseling, it's this: To make lasting changes, you've got to believe that what you're getting is loads better than what you're giving up. What's worked for my clients is doing some self-exploration to arrive at a place where the pros of changing truly outweigh the cons—not because they *think* that's where they should be, but because they believe it!

I once had a client who told me she'd never understood those people who'd *really* rather have an apple and almonds than a few Oreos. She always thought they were lying or had an iron will when they'd pass on (free!) goodies at work and eat the healthy foods they'd brought instead. Then, one Monday afternoon, she was reaching for the candy dish when it hit her. She'd spent the last week eating healthy foods and had been able to join her family on a bike ride. For the first time in a long time, they hadn't gone without her. The satisfaction she got from that bike ride meant more than the momentary satisfaction the chocolate would provide. In that instant, she really did want a crisp apple and not that handful of M&M's. And her choice had nothing to do with willpower. —*Cynthia*

6. GET CENTERED—SELF-CENTERED. Before you go any further, I want you to grab a pencil and fill in the blanks.

Below, write the names of the most important people in your life.

_____

_____

_____

_____

_____

When you have completed your list, turn to the next page in this book. *Don't turn the page until you have completed this list.*

DID YOU KNOW ?

Your blood pressure level is likely to be higher in winter than in summer. Scientists think cold weather may cause blood vessels to narrow, constricting blood flow.

Okay. Did you put yourself at the top of your own list? Are you even *on* your list? My guess is that if you *did* include yourself, you were dead last. And that's not surprising, because most women are so *other-directed* that they completely overlook their own happiness and needs. If I asked you about your relationship with your husband or your parents or your children, no doubt you could give me specific, detailed, layered answers. But if I asked you to describe how you treat yourself, how different would the answer be?

When you're trying to change a behavior (particularly a health-oriented behavior like eating better and exercising more), it's absolutely essential to learn to put yourself first. After all, what is a diet if not a contract between you and yourself? You have chosen to read and follow the principles of the *Flat Belly Diet*. I presume you've done this for the sake of how you look, how you feel, and how your health measures up. And while you've made a commitment to stay on the food plan—it's far more than that. It's a commitment to put yourself at the top of the agenda, to recognize that you are special and you deserve the time, energy, and effort that's equal to everything else in your life.

Now I want you to find a nice sheet of clean, crisp note paper and rewrite the list of the most important people in your life. This time put yourself at the top, where you rightfully belong. Post the list someplace you'll see it often, like on your mirror or the refrigerator door. You'll be amazed how much less stressful life is when you remember to always look out for Number One.

7. GET IT ON THE CALENDAR. Now that you have placed yourself at the top of the list, acknowledge that "me" time is not an indulgence but an *essential* factor in your health and happiness, not to mention your success on the *Flat Belly Diet*. "Me" time is yours to take, if you're willing to say, "This is *my* moment, and it takes priority over everything else." How about starting with 15 minutes a day?

I know what you're thinking: *Hey, Liz, I don't have 15 minutes!* You're wrong, and I'm going to prove it to you. On the first 4 days of this plan, I'm going to ask you to take 2 to 3 minutes before every meal to focus on yourself, your ultimate goal, and how much you can achieve when you put your mind to it. I call these little exercises Mind Tricks because they're simple tasks that help wake up your brain and draw your attention to the act of eating. If you can manage a few minutes before every meal, you've found your 15 minutes.

SASS FROM SASS

"Just Say No Way to Trans Fat."

I'm a firm believer in eating fat, but in creating this plan, I was adamant that a certain type of fat be excluded altogether: trans fatty acids, or trans fat. These man-made fats are created from vegetable oils in a process called partial hydrogenation, which adds hydrogen to liquid unsaturated oils. This changes their structure into a form that helps hold ingredients together in foods like pie crusts, cookies, or crackers. Because trans fats spoil more slowly, they extend a product's shelf life. Research shows that not only are trans fats bad for your heart because they clog arteries and raise "bad" LDL cholesterol, but they also increase the accumulation of belly fat, according to research conducted at Wake Forest University. To avoid trans fat, look at the Nutrition Facts panel, and check the ingredient list. Labels are allowed to list trans fat as zero grams if they contain less than half a gram per serving. If the word *hydrogenated* appears in the ingredient list, limit or avoid the food—even if it says "zero grams of trans fat."

—*Cynthia*

As you continue past the 4th day on the *Flat Belly Diet*, I'll discuss the importance of keeping a journal. Every day, I'll give you another exercise in reflection—something I call a Core Confidence. These exercises will help focus each day's journal entry and give you a theme to discuss on the page. And guess what? *Each one takes about 15 minutes.* (Don't you love when that happens?)

Armed and Ready: The Big Three Questions

Now you understand the scientific underpinnings of both emotional eating and the body's physiological response to stress. And you can now master the unique forces at work in the mind-belly connection. You're also equipped with seven useful stress-busting strategies that will help you manage the stress in your life during this journey of healthy eating.

But before we embark on the first part of the *Flat Belly Diet*—the Four-Day Anti-Bloat Jumpstart—I want you to take a few moments to reflect on these three vital change-related questions.

1. *Who am I doing this for?*

    There is only one acceptable answer to this question, and that is "me"—and no one else. You're probably a lot more comfortable doing things for others, but

Why do I have to keep a food journal?

The food journal serves several functions. First, food journals raise your awareness about exactly what and how much you're eating. Research also tells us that dieters benefit from accountability, particularly when they're starting out on a new plan. Writing in a journal each day will help you stay committed to your goals, keep your behaviors on track, and lead you to better results.

how often do you really do something for yourself? Losing weight, if you need to, is really the ultimate expression of self-caring, more so than booking the occasional massage or regular mani-pedi. That's because losing weight now, especially if you're overweight or obese, can make the difference between feeling tired and feeling energized. It can mean the difference between a retirement you'll enjoy and one plagued by health problems like diabetes or heart disease. As I noted before, the fat in your belly is the most dangerous and deadly. Choosing to cure yourself—especially with a plan like this that promises not just weight loss but also a whole host of other health benefits—may be the greatest gift you can give yourself.

2. *How can I make the next 32 days easier?*

Think *Flat Belly* feng shui. I'm not talking about moving your refrigerator into the basement or hanging a mirror over your stove. I'm simply suggesting that you consider all the ways you can make your office and home surroundings more supportive of your new goal. That means divesting the pantry and refrigerator of tempting food or keeping all the junk food in the second cabinet from the left. As for your office, you may want to clean out your "junk" drawer. That "emergency" candy stash isn't going to do you any favors. And now is the time to scope out a place to put your Snack Pack.

3. *Who's on Team Me?*

Before you begin, consider having a serious heart-to-heart with everyone in your immediate circle. Tell them why you're doing this, why it's so important to you, what you need from them, and how you think it might affect your relationship. You might need to swap your family's Sunday IHOP stop with a healthier breakfast at home, or happy hour with the girls for a cup of tea at a local café. When they realize how important this is to you, they'll listen, and I'll bet some of them will even want to join in!

READ A FLAT BELLY
SUCCESS
STORY

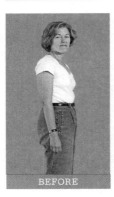

BEFORE

AFTER

Kathy Brechner

AGE: 53

POUNDS LOST:

5

IN 32 DAYS

ALL-OVER
INCHES LOST:

7.5

"

I REALLY DIDN'T HAVE ALL THAT MUCH WEIGHT TO LOSE," Kathy Brechner says. "Only 5 pounds, actually. But believe me, they were the *toughest* 5 pounds I've ever tried to get off in my life." She credited much of the difficulty in losing this weight to the fact that she's 53 and hovering near menopause. But her current lifestyle wasn't helping, either. "I serve as a volunteer to our local board of education, so I'm often on the run. I'm eating in the car half the time, eating late at night, not exercising enough, running the kids around to their activities in between. Something had to give."

Kathy was concerned that "something" would be her health because, as she points out, she has a family history of heart disease, type 2 diabetes, and high blood pressure. And so, with the image in the back of her mind of the number on the scale slowly creeping up, and knowing that at this point in her life she was facing the same fate as her parents, she realized it was time to see what new steps she might take to improve on what she was already doing—particularly since what she was doing simply wasn't working.

That was when she learned about the *Flat Belly Diet* and its focus on good health as well as weight loss. She was already familiar with the benefits of eating MUFAs and the healthy style of

Mediterranean-type foods. But she felt she needed more structure. "I think that was the initial attraction," she explains. "I just liked the idea of the 32-day principle. I knew I could do anything for 32 days, so why not give it a try?"

She says the diet completely changed how she and her family view portions. "My husband looked at the menu I had chosen for one of our dinners and said, *'One-eighth cup of pasta? Who can get by on $1/_8$ cup of pasta?'* But we not only could—we did. For snacks, I have a flat wicker tray on the counter, and I have small dishes of the different nuts sitting there. A measuring spoon is right next to it because it's just too easy to grab handfuls and scarf them down before you know it. The diet has even covered the 'quick grab' for nights when I have meetings. I could have a prepared meal and know I was giving something healthy to my family and still sticking to the diet."

Is she happy with her results? "I'm ecstatic!" she says. "The *Flat Belly Diet* brought me to the goal I set out to achieve: 5 pounds—gone. For the first time. And as a bonus, my energy level is so much higher than it's been in the past. I'm not getting any more sleep. I haven't been doing any additional exercise. So it has to be what I'm eating." She adds, "I think every woman at or approaching menopause should know this: There's never a better time to start thinking about your health than *right now*. Keeping your weight down and your energy up gets harder as you age, so why not be a little ahead of that curve?"

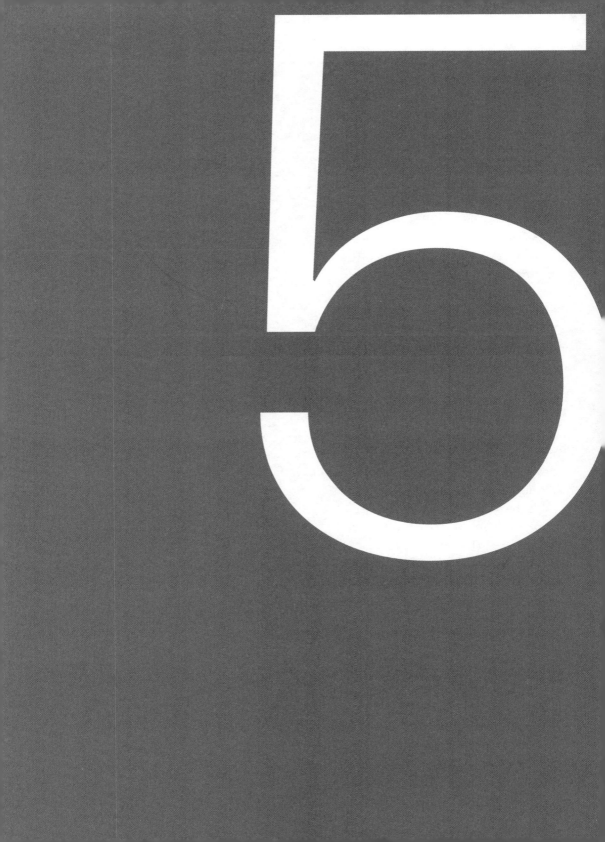

THE FOUR-DAY ANTI-BLOAT JUMPSTART

THIS CHAPTER IS A DREAM COME TRUE for any woman who's ever suffered from a bloated belly. A number of factors influence how puffy you feel on any given day, including what you eat and how you take care of yourself. But this chapter will help you address your bloating—whatever its cause—immediately. In just 4 days, you'll lose several pounds and inches, which will start a cascade of motivation and energy that will immediately set you up for success on the rest of the plan.

I was in my twenties when I first really understood the phenomenon of water retention. I was a magazine editor in Cleveland at the time, and every Friday morning, the staff met at 9 a.m. sharp in a big new conference room on the far side of the floor. It was in that room that I noticed that my engagement ring always seemed to mysteriously fit more snugly.

Once I noticed the connection between the mysterious poof and a particular day and time, I started paying a little more attention to what I ate and drank the rest of the week. And then I realized what was happening: Thursday was pizza night. Every week, I'd meet my then-fiancé, Steve, for a pie at Mama Santa's in Little Italy. *And I'd salt every slice.*

Bloating can really ruin a girl's day, not to mention her confidence. That's why the *Flat Belly Diet* starts with a Four-Day Anti-Bloat Jumpstart Plan. This phase will start a cascade of confidence because it promises to shrink your belly—a loss of up to $5^3/_4$ total inches—in just 4 short days. How do I know? Because we tested the entire *Flat Belly Diet*—including the Jumpstart—on women just like you, holding weigh-ins on a biweekly basis. You're reading their stories throughout this book, and you can find more by visiting **flatbellydiet.com**. More than half of our test panel lost at least 1 full inch from their bellies during the Jumpstart period.

There's nothing more satisfying and confidence-boosting when you're starting a new eating plan than being able to see—almost immediately—your pants get-

DID YOU KNOW ?

The word *metabolism* refers to the number of calories you burn per day. Some of that comes from the energy your cells use to perform everyday lifesaving functions (like maintaining heart muscle contractions that keep your blood flowing). That's called your basal metabolic rate. You also burn calories through activity, whether that's taking out the garbage or running a 5-K. The last piece of the metabolism puzzle comes from digesting your food, which burns calories. This is called the "thermic effect" of food. The sum of all the calories you burn (basal + activity + digestion) equals your total metabolism, or total metabolic rate.

Being less active affects your metabolism in two ways: It makes the second "plus" in this equation smaller, but you also lose muscle, which reduces the basal number in the equation.

ting looser, your cheekbones getting more noticeable, your muscles getting more defined. It inspires commitment and a desire to succeed. And that's what I want for you to get out of this book more than anything else: success.

The Four-Day Anti-Bloat Jumpstart Plan has been created for the very specific purpose of eliminating gas, heavy solids, and excess fluid so you will quickly feel and look lighter. Bear in mind: This is *not* a wacky—and dangerous—"detox" plan. You'll be eating whole fruits, vegetables, and grains and fresh, naturally flavored water—wholesome food prepared in simple, delicious ways. In fact, it's what you *won't* be eating and drinking and doing that really makes the Jumpstart so effective. To see how, I think it helps to first understand how your digestive system works.

Digestion 101

YOUR GASTROINTESTINAL (GI) tract is about 35 feet long from top to bottom. Read that again: *35 feet long!* That's about seven of you, lying end to end. And it's all coiled up inside your torso (along with most of your major organs and, yes, belly fat). That's why, when your GI tract is irritated or in any way dysfunctional, it greatly impacts how you feel overall. But before we talk about potential problems, let's go over the basics.

The primary role of your GI tract is to extract essential nutrients like carbohydrates, proteins, fats, vitamins, minerals, and water from the food you eat and the beverages you drink. These nutrients are transported through the walls of the small and large intestines into the bloodstream, where they're then distributed to wherever they're needed. For instance, when you eat a turkey sandwich, your GI tract breaks it down into bits of carbohydrate (the bread and vegetables), protein (the turkey), fat (the mayo), fiber (from the bread), and all sorts of vitamins and minerals. Carbohydrates, protein, and fat get broken down even further into sugars, amino acids, and fatty acids, respectively. The sugars go to fuel brain and muscle activity (not to mention the doings of every cell in your body), the amino acids get used to build muscle and bone, and the fats get stored for future energy needs or get used to manufacture hormones and other essential compounds.

Ultimately, hundreds of biochemical reactions occur, and the chemical end products of that turkey sandwich have thousands of uses. But you can see that the ultimate job of your digestive system is to extract as much nutrition as possible out of everything you put in your mouth.

The whole process starts with saliva. Saliva contains digestive enzymes that help break the chemical bonds holding foods together so they can be easily crushed and macerated by your teeth. These enzymes are pretty fast-acting; if you put a cracker or piece of toast on your tongue, you'll notice it quickly breaking down, even before you start to chew. Your tongue helps position the food in your mouth and moves it toward the back of your throat toward your esophagus, the 10-inch connector between your mouth and your stomach. It's different from your windpipe, or trachea, which connects your mouth to your lungs. When you swallow, a little flap called the epiglottis covers the opening of the trachea to guard against choking. (If you've ever had food "go down the wrong way," it's because your epiglottis didn't cover your trachea quickly enough.)

Once in the esophagus, rhythmic automatic muscle contractions help push the food toward your stomach. There, acids further break down your meal, while your stomach muscles churn the whole mixture into what amounts to a nutrient-dense puree, which is then pushed into the 22-foot-long tunnel that is your small intestine. There, with the help of bile, a fat emulsifier produced by your gallbladder, and additional enzymes produced by your pancreas, your meal

If I eat a pound of food, will I gain a pound of weight?

A half-gallon of water weighs 4 pounds, but if you drink a half-gallon of water, you won't gain 4 pounds of fat. You will, however, temporarily weigh 4 pounds more on the scale—that is, until your kidneys eliminate that water. That's because when you step on that scale, you are weighing anything that has weight to it—the water you just drank, the undigested food you ate a few hours ago, the waste from the food you ate yesterday that hasn't worked its way all the way through your GI tract yet, your muscle, skeleton, your body fat, and the clothes you're wearing (if any).

Most of the weight fluctuations we see on a scale have to do with our fluid status, because that's the variable that changes the most from hour to hour and day to day. If you're retaining water, you could easily weigh 5 pounds more, and if you're dehydrated (maybe from being sick), you could weigh 5 pounds less. Changes in actual body fat, however, happen much slower and are controlled solely by calories. It takes an excess of 3,500 calories (that means above and beyond the calories you burn) to create 1 pound of body fat. If you ate 700 calories more than your body could burn in 1 day, you'd gain $1/5$ of a pound. Do that 5 days in a row starting on a Monday, and by the end of the workweek, you've accumulated 1 pound of fat. (By the way, a pound of fat is nothing to sneeze at; it's equal to 4 sticks of butter!) So, while that number staring back at you seems to jump up and down like a yo-yo, you can see that it really takes several days in a row of overeating to even gain 1 pound of actual body fat. The scale is much less fickle when it comes to fat than water!

is absorbed through the walls of your intestine into your bloodstream in the form of individual nutrient building blocks—sugars, fatty acids, and amino acids from carbohydrates, fats, and proteins, respectively. Vitamins and minerals are also absorbed during the journey through the small intestine.

You may have noticed that I didn't mention dietary fiber. That's because you don't absorb fiber. Fiber fills you up, but doesn't add to your overall caloric intake. While fiber does contain as many calories as any other form of carbohydrate—about 4 per gram—your body isn't able to use them for energy. Instead, fiber just moves through your body nearly intact. Along the way, it binds to cholesterol, helping to shuttle it out of your system. A few studies have also found that fiber can prevent absorption of other calories you consume—up to 90 per day.

All the nutrients that do enter the bloodstream travel straight to the liver, which filters out wastes and decides where everything usable should go. Anything that isn't absorbed—fiber, waste by-products—travels down into the large intestine and finally through the colon and rectum. Before it leaves your body, small amounts of water and minerals are absorbed in a last-ditch effort to extract every last drop of importance out of that turkey sandwich.

Now that you're familiar with your GI tract, let's take a closer look at what's going on when you feel like a beach ball has taken up residence there.

Gas, Solids & Liquids: The Balloon Gang

THINK OF ONE of those very long, narrow balloons that you find at a child's birthday party, the ones that clowns twist into different shapes. That balloon represents your GI tract. Now picture the balloon filled with water, air, or solid food. Each of these substances expands the balloon but does so in a different way.

■ AIR: When air enters the intestine—say, for example, from chewing gum, talking, drinking carbonated beverages, or even smoking—it doesn't get absorbed into the bloodstream. Instead, it remains trapped until it can be

DID YOU KNOW ?

A calorie is a unit of energy needed to increase the temperature of 1 gram of water by 1°C. In everyday terms, it's energy that can have one of four origins and one of three destinations. There are four sources of calories: carbohydrates, protein, fat, and alcohol. The first three types are essential to the body, but alcohol is not. When one of these types becomes available to the body, the cells will do one of three things with this energy. Basically, there is a priority system.

Fuel is the number one priority of every cell in the body. Just like cars need gasoline, cells need fuel to perform their jobs (breathing, circulation, movement, etc.). Carbohydrate calories are the cells' preferred source of energy. The next priority is repair, healing, and maintenance. Your body takes the energy from proteins and fats and uses them to patch up cells that are damaged or create new cells. Your muscles, bones, skin, and immune system rely on protein and fat energy for this work. Finally, if all the cells are properly fueled and repaired or replaced, your body takes the leftover or unneeded energy and stores it away in your fat cells.

When your body is in "energy balance," it means the number of calories that showed up for work (the amount eaten) matched your needs perfectly. If you're in a positive energy balance, too many showed up, and you end up storing some (i.e., weight gain); a negative energy balance means not enough calories are available. This can result in fatigue, feeling run-down, and getting sick or injured. The *Flat Belly Diet* is designed to keep you in balance—it provides enough energy in the form of carbohydrates, proteins, and fats, but not too much.

eventually expelled via a belch or flatulence. Until then, it meanders through your GI tract, causing distension and discomfort.

■ SOLID: It's generally just a matter of time before solid food gets broken down and absorbed or expelled. But until then, you're feeling like a beached whale.

■ LIQUID: Just like solid foods, liquid eventually gets absorbed, but sometimes we retain more fluid than our body really needs.

The Four Bad Guys of Bloat

THE FOUR-DAY ANTI-BLOAT Jumpstart has been created for the very specific purpose of eliminating gas, heavy solids, and excess fluid so you will almost instantly feel and look lighter. Before we move on to the nitty-gritty details of the plan—what and when you'll eat—I want to explain four lifestyle factors that can also influence how prone you are to bloating or fluid retention.

1. STRESS: It triggers a complex sequence of hormonal fluctuations that raise blood pressure and divert blood to your extremities, where energy is most needed. This process allows you to run faster or lift more if necessary, but it also causes your digestive system to slow down significantly, which means you absorb nutrients more slowly (and sometimes miss some). As a result of the slowdown, your last meal may stick around in your intestine, causing bloat.

2. LACK OF FLUID: You've probably heard you need about eight glasses of water a day. Drinking water and even eating "watery" foods like melon, greens, and other fruits and vegetables has enormous health benefits, including warding off fatigue, maintaining your body's proper fluid balance, and guarding against water retention and constipation, which can cause bloating. Eight glasses is just a guideline; everyone's fluid needs vary according to activity level and body. Although all fluids (and water-packed foods) count toward your overall fluid intake, not all of these are permitted on the Four-Day Anti-Bloat Jumpstart.

3. LACK OF SLEEP: Too little sleep disrupts the intricate workings of your nervous system, which controls the rhythmic contractions of your GI tract and helps keep things humming along. It also affects your overall ability to manage and cope with stress. It's important to get at least 7 hours of sleep a night. If you have trouble sleeping, consult a sleep expert, or visit the National Sleep Foundation's Web site at sleepfoundation.org.

4. AIR TRAVEL: The average plane maintains cabin pressure equal to 5,000 to 8,000 feet above sea level in order to provide a comfortable atmosphere for the passengers. At that altitude, free air in the body cavities tends to expand by around 25 percent.[1] Pressure changes also increase the production of gases in your GI tract. As the pressure in the cabin drops, the air in your intestines expands, causing bloating and discomfort. Cabin pressurization is also responsible for increased water retention because it impacts your body's natural fluid balance. Add in the dehydration caused by recirculated air and those bloat miles add up. Your best defense is to drink as much water as possible before and during your flight and to walk around as often as possible.

A Thinner, Lighter You in Four Days!

THE FOUR-DAY ANTI-BLOAT Jumpstart literally abolishes the foods, beverages, and behaviors that cause your belly to pooch out. And—as a bonus—it provides guidelines for reducing the chances of ever feeling this way again. As you experience this phase, remember that you're taking the first step of your journey toward a healthier lifestyle. It's not just a smaller dress size. Here's what you're really gaining:

- An easy, safe, food-based solution for the body part you most want to change
- A more intense focus on your long-term health
- A reduced risk of heart disease, diabetes, and cancer
- A comprehensive understanding of what constitutes a healthy meal
- A more mindful approach to meals that virtually eliminates emotional eating

Remember: This Four-Day Anti-Bloat Jumpstart is designed to eliminate both bloating and water retention. Losing bloat is not the same as burning fat (we'll tackle that in the next chapter!), but it still creates a major change in your appearance and confidence level.

That's not to say you won't lose some serious pounds! And you'll start right now. If you follow the instructions provided for the next 4 days, we estimate that you can expect to lose as much as 7 pounds and up to $5^3/_4$ inches from your waist, hips, thighs, bust, and arms combined. *No sweat necessary.* That's right—no exercise is needed. I didn't make these numbers up. They are actual pounds

(continued on page 76)

ARE YOU PRONE TO BELLY BLOAT?

DISCOVER HOW SUSCEPTIBLE YOU ARE TO BELLY BLOAT AND WATER RETENTION BY TAKING THIS SIMPLE QUIZ. WHEN YOU'RE FINISHED, ADD UP YOUR SCORE AND COMPARE IT TO THE RATINGS ON THE OPPOSITE PAGE.

QUESTION	A	B
Do you tend to eat too quickly? If **yes**, add 1 point for every speedy meal you eat per day (e.g., if you eat 4 times a day and they're all eaten at rapid speed, put a 4 in column A). If **no**, place a 1 in column B.		
Do you believe you are lactose intolerant? If **yes**, place a 1 in column A. If **no**, place a 1 in column B.		
Do you tend to talk a lot while you eat? If **yes**, place a 1 in column A. If **no**, place a 1 in column B.		
Do you add table salt to your food? If **yes**, add 1 point for every salt-sprinkled meal you eat per day (e.g., if you eat 4 times a day and you salt each meal, put a 4 in column A). If **no**, place a 1 in column B.		
Do you regularly binge on carbs? In other words, do you have episodes of eating more than you usually would of carb-rich foods at least once a week? If **yes**, add 1 point for every high-carb binge you can recall over the past week. If **no**, place a 1 in column B.		
Add 1 point to column A for each of the following foods you eat at least once a week: beans, lentils, nuts, cauliflower, broccoli, Brussels sprouts, cabbage, onions, peppers, raw citrus fruits. If you don't eat any of these foods at least once a week, add a 1 to column B.		
Do you chew gum, including sugarless? If **yes**, add 1 point for every piece of gum you chew per week (e.g., if you chew 1 piece a day, put a 7 in column A). If **no**, place a 1 in column B.		
Do you use sugar substitutes? If **yes**, add 1 point for every packet you use per day (e.g., if you use 2 in your morning coffee, place a 2 in column A). If **no**, place a 1 in column B.		
Do you eat sugar-free candies or sweets? If **yes**, add 1 point for every serving of sugar-free food you eat per week (e.g., if you suck on sugar-free candies in the afternoon at work M–F, place a 5 in column A). If **no**, place a 1 in column B.		
Do you suffer from sleep apnea? If **yes**, add 1 point. If **no**, place a 1 in column B.		
Do you eat fried foods? If **yes**, add 1 point for every serving of fried foods you eat per week (e.g., if you treat yourself to fries only once a week, place a 1 in column A). If **no**, place a 1 in column B.		

QUESTION	A	B
Do you drink carbonated beverages? If **yes**, add 1 point for every can or bottle you drink per week (e.g., if you drink 2 diet colas a day, place a 14 in column A). If **no**, place a 1 in column B.		
Do you drink coffee, tea, or acidic juice (orange or tomato) daily? If **yes**, add 1 point for every glass or mug you drink per week (e.g., if you drink 2 cups of coffee a day, place a 14 in column B). If **no**, place a 1 in column B.		
Would you rate your everyday stress level as high? If **yes**, place a 1 in column A. If **no**, place a 1 in column B.		
Add up your score in each column:	*TOTAL* from column A:	*TOTAL* from column B:

FINAL TOTAL (Subtract B score from A score): _____

IF YOU SCORED:

A NEGATIVE NUMBER: Congratulations! Your bloating risk is relatively low. You're already avoiding a lot of the foods and bad habits that contribute to excessive bloating and water retention. But that doesn't mean the Four-Day Anti-Bloat Jumpstart won't help you. You may not lose significant inches, but you will still *feel* lighter and healthier and be on a better path to long-term well-being.

0–5: NOT SO BAD. You probably experience come-and-go bloat. It's what I like to call bloat-flow—one day you're swollen; a few days later, you've deflated again. The good news is that you can tame your tummy without making too many changes to your lifestyle. You should get some immediate gratification on the Four-Day Anti-Bloat Jumpstart.

5–10: You may experience a little withdrawal from your usual habits, but you'll be handsomely rewarded—you should experience a noticeable difference after just 2 days on the Jumpstart.

10+: Congratulations again! If you're confused, don't be. I say congratulations because you are perfectly suited to seeing fantastic results on the Four-Day Anti-Bloat Jumpstart, so you're virtually primed for success on the *Flat Belly Diet* as a whole. The Jumpstart itself is really a cleansing—of foods, drinks, and behaviors—that cause your body to unnecessarily hang on to fluid or produce excess gas and waste. It's not a detox but a cleaner, simpler way to eat than you may be used to. And because of that, you're likely to see some major belly shrinkage.

When Bloating Gets Bad

Bloating is a common condition, but in some cases, it can be a sign of a more serious health problem. It's time to see a doctor when:

- Your symptoms don't improve on the Four-Day Anti-Bloat Jumpstart.
- You're suffering from chronic constipation, diarrhea, nausea, or vomiting.
- You have persistent abdominal or rectal pain or heartburn.
- You've lost weight without trying.
- You have a fever you can't explain.
- There is blood in your urine.

lost, all calculated by an expert who weighed and measured our test panelists. Rest assured: This plan has been proven to work on real women just like you.

Four Days—What to Avoid

■ THE SALT SHAKER, SALT-BASED SEASONINGS, AND HIGHLY PRO-CESSED FOODS: Water is attracted to sodium, so when you take in higher than usual amounts of sodium, you'll temporarily retain more fluid—which contributes to a sluggish feeling, a puffy appearance, and extra water weight. Cutting back on sodium and boosting your water intake will help bring your body back into balance. It'll also help reduce your risks of hypertension and osteoporosis. If you find your food lacks flavor without a few shakes of salt, use the recommended salt-free seasonings.

■ EXCESS CARBS: As a backup energy source, your muscles store a type of carbohydrate called glycogen. Every gram of glycogen is stored with about 3 grams of water. But unless you're running a marathon tomorrow, you don't need all this stockpiled fuel. Decrease your intake of high-carbohydrate foods such as pasta, bananas, bagels, and pretzels to temporarily train your body to access this stored fuel and burn it off. At the same time, you'll be getting rid of all that excess stored fluid.

■ BULKY RAW FOODS: **A half-cup serving of cooked carrots delivers the same nutrition as 1 cup raw, but it takes up less room in your GI tract. Eat only cooked vegetables, smaller portions of unsweetened dried fruit, and canned fruits in natural juice. This will allow you to meet your nutrient needs without expanding your GI tract with extra volume.**

■ GASSY FOODS: **Certain foods simply create more gas in your GI tract. They include legumes, cauliflower, broccoli, Brussels sprouts, cabbage, onions, peppers, and citrus fruits.**

■ CHEWING GUM: **You probably don't realize this, but when you chew gum, you swallow air. All that air gets trapped in your GI tract and causes pressure, bloating, and belly expansion.**

■ SUGAR ALCOHOLS: **These sugar substitutes, which go by the names xylitol or maltitol, are often found in low-calorie or low-carb products like cookies, candy, and energy bars because they taste sweet. Like fiber, your GI tract can't absorb most of them. That's good for your calorie bottom line but not so good for your belly. Sugar alcohols cause gas, abdominal distention, bloating, and diarrhea. Avoid them.**

■ FRIED FOODS: **Fatty foods, especially the fried variety, are digested more slowly, causing you to feel heavy and bloated.**

■ SPICY FOODS: **Foods seasoned with black pepper, nutmeg, cloves,**

DID YOU KNOW?

One way to take up less space in your stomach is to be mindful of what you put into it. For example, 1 cup of grapes takes up four times as much space as eating ¼ cup of unsweetened raisins.

chili powder, hot sauces, onions, garlic, mustard, chili, barbecue sauce, horse-radish, catsup, tomato sauce, or vinegar can all stimulate the release of stomach acid, which can cause irritation.

■ CARBONATED DRINKS: **Where do you think all those bubbles end up? They gang up in your belly!**

■ ALCOHOL, COFFEE, TEA, HOT COCOA, AND ACIDIC FRUIT JUICES: Each of these high-acid beverages can irritate your GI tract, causing swelling.

Four Days—What to Do

■ FOLLOW THE FOUR-DAY PLAN EXACTLY. **This includes four smaller meals, one of which is a refreshing smoothie. This reduces the amount of food in your digestive system at any one time, cuts back on the release of stomach acids, and gets your body used to a four-meal-a-day schedule (which you'll be following on the rest of the *Flat Belly Diet*).**

■ EAT FOUR MEALS A DAY. **The Jumpstart includes fewer calories—about 1,200 daily—than you'll be eating on the *Flat Belly Diet*, which allows about 1,600 per day. Eating less for these 4 days reduces the amount of food in your GI tract at any one time, cuts back on the release of stomach acids, and gets your body used to a four-meal-a-day schedule.**

You'll notice a few staples, including sunflower seeds, flaxseed oil, string cheese, and carrots. There are three reasons you'll see these items appear repeatedly. First, we tried to limit the amount of food you have to buy to get started—and ensure you'll eat it before it goes bad. Second, we wanted to deliver a lot of nutritional and bloat-free bang for the buck. Finally, we chose foods that need no added salt or condiments to taste good, so you won't be tempted to reach for one of these potential bloat-promoters.

■ TAKE A QUICK 5-MINUTE AFTER-MEAL WALK. **Moving your body helps release air that has been trapped in your GI tract, relieving pressure and**

I am very prone to water retention. I'm drawn to salty foods more than sweet ones, and whenever I have an especially salty treat (movie popcorn, anyone?), I get "puffy" for at least a day after. So if I have an early morning TV appearance, I'm extra careful about what I eat the night before—you can bet there's no soy sauce involved! Some of us are genetically more prone to this phenomenon than others—nothing you can do about that. Here are some things to keep in mind about water retention, whether it's been a regular companion or occasional nuisance for you.

Remember, it's not fat! I once had a friend call me in a panic saying she'd gained 4 pounds in one day. I asked if she'd eaten all her usual meals plus an extra 14,000 calories—because that, my friends, is what you'd need to eat to gain 4 pounds of body fat in a day. She hadn't been bingeing, and I'm guessing you don't, either. So don't beat yourself up about that kind of weight gain. It's just water retention, and you'll lose it again.

Know your own body. Keeping a journal can help you track certain patterns. You might be more prone to water retention during a certain part of your menstrual cycle, and journaling will show you when and for how long you tend to hang on to that extra fluid.

Plan ahead. If you're going to be in your bathing suit or you just plain want to look your leanest, avoid salty foods for at least several days ahead of time. This is one kind of weight change you can control completely.   —*Cynthia*

bloating. All it takes is a leisurely stroll around the block, inside your office building, or at the mall; a quick walk with your dog, a neighbor, or your family members after dinner—anything that gets you moving for just 5 minutes. You can walk for longer if you like, but at least 5 minutes are needed to help get things moving inside your belly.

■ DRINK ONE ENTIRE RECIPE OF CYNTHIA'S REFRESHING SIGNATURE SASSY WATER EVERY DAY. We call it Sassy because it's a heck of a lot perkier than plain old water, just like Cynthia herself! But the ingredients in here aren't just for flavor: The ginger also helps calm and soothe your GI tract. Even more important: The simple act of making this Sassy Water every day will serve as a reminder for these 4 days that life is a little bit different, that things are going to change. It will keep you focused on the flat-belly task ahead.

SASSY WATER

2 liters water (about 8½ cups)
1 teaspoon freshly grated ginger root
1 medium cucumber, peeled and thinly sliced
1 medium lemon, thinly sliced
12 mint leaves

Combine all ingredients in a large pitcher, chill in the refrigerator, and let flavors blend overnight.

■ EAT SLOWLY. Often, when you eat quickly, you take in large gulps of air without realizing it. All that excess air gets trapped in your digestive system and causes bloating (think of a balloon stretched to capacity). Taking your time will help prevent the expansion. It will also keep you calm, and allow you to connect with the concept of mealtime as a moment to stop, rest, and reflect. Too often, we hurry through meals, always trying to get to the next block of time on our to-do schedule. Let's put an end to this for these 4 days, and beyond, and remember the joy that comes from respecting mealtime.

■ WORK YOUR MIND. The first days of a diet are never easy, and these 4 days are no exception. I'm asking you to change how you eat and to give up some of the foods you're used to eating or drinking—and perhaps imagine you can't live without. Of course, it's going to be worth it in the end—it does work, and you will see your belly shrink. But until you see that poof disappear, you'll need a mental tune-up. That's where my Mind Tricks come in.

Mind Tricks are a way of giving a meal importance—making it a special, you-focused moment. They'll help you stay mindful of what you're eating and why.

Your Four-Day Shopping List

PRODUCE
☐ 2 pints grape tomatoes
☐ 1 pint fresh or frozen green beans
☐ 2 large red potatoes
☐ 10 oz bag baby carrots
☐ Half pint cremini mushrooms
☐ 1 large yellow squash
☐ 4 medium cucumbers
☐ 4 medium lemons

DAIRY
☐ ½ gallon lactose-free skim milk
☐ 1 package low-fat string cheese

FROZEN FOODS
☐ 10 oz bag frozen unsweetened blueberries
☐ 10 oz bag frozen unsweetened peaches
☐ 10 oz bag frozen unsweetened strawberries

DRY GOODS
☐ 12 oz box unsweetened corn flakes
☐ 12 oz box Rice Krispies®
☐ 12 oz box instant Cream of Wheat®
☐ 14 oz box instant brown rice
☐ 24 oz jar unsweetened applesauce
☐ 8 oz can pineapple tidbits canned in pineapple juice
☐ 1 cup bulk (or 1 small package) roasted or raw unsalted sunflower seeds

☐ 8 oz bottle cold-pressed organic flaxseed oil
☐ 8 oz bottle olive oil
☐ 15 oz package raisins
☐ 7 oz container dried plums

SPICES
☐ 1–2 knuckles fresh ginger root
☐ 2 bunches fresh mint

MEAT/SEAFOOD
☐ 2 packages organic deli turkey
☐ ¼ pound tilapia
☐ ⅓ pound boneless skinless chicken breast
☐ ¼ pound turkey breast cutlet
☐ 3 oz can chunk light tuna in water

ANY OF THESE APPROVED SALT-FREE SEASONINGS
☐ Original and Italian medley Mrs. Dash® salt-free seasoning blends
☐ Fresh or dried: basil, bay leaf, cinnamon, curry powder, dill, ginger, lemon or lime juice, marjoram, mint, oregano, paprika, pepper, rosemary, sage, tarragon, or thyme
☐ Aged balsamic vinegar

As you embark on the 4 days' worth of Mind Tricks—16 in all, one at every meal—you'll surely find some that are so appealing that you'll want to repeat them again and again. In fact, you should repeat your favorites until they become a ritual. I'm all for doing whatever it takes to make you feel special.

Track Your Progress

STUDIES HAVE CONTINUALLY shown that keeping a log of what you eat and how you feel while you're eating helps you stay on track with new lifestyle choices. There is now increasing evidence to support the concept that journaling has a positive impact on physical well-being. University of Texas at Austin researcher James Pennebaker, PhD, has scientifically shown that regular journaling strengthens immune cells called T-lymphocytes.[2] Other research indicates that journaling may help decrease the symptoms of asthma and rheumatoid arthritis. Pennebaker believes that writing about stressful events helps you come to terms with them, thus reducing the impact of these stressors on your physical health.

But in addition to all those things, keeping a journal is a simple way to feel as if you're making significant progress. When I was training for a marathon, one of the biggest motivators in getting me into my running shoes and out the door

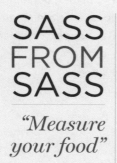

SASS FROM SASS

"Measure your food"

Always measure foods—especially those that pack a lot of calories in small amounts, including oil, nuts, seeds, peanut butter, avocado, pasta, rice, and oatmeal. Measuring will help ensure that this carefully calculated plan gives you the results you're looking for. Without measuring, it's very easy to miscalculate and rack up hundreds of extra calories. I've certainly seen this in my practice as a registered dietitian.   —*Cynthia*

every morning was my running log. All I wanted to do was fill that baby up, and I would get engrossed in watching the mileage accumulate week after week. Similarly, a journal will inspire you to focus on and achieve your weight loss goals.

For the Four-Day Anti-Bloat Jumpstart, your journal is incorporated into your meal plan. Later, when you complete the Jumpstart and begin the *Flat Belly Diet*, I'll ask you to spend a bit more time journaling about specific issues that you may have about food and your body confidence. For now, take these 4 days to get used to the format of the food journal—and start building the habit of sitting down and recording everything you've put into your mouth that day.

A few rules of the journaling journey:

1. Forget spelling and punctuation.
2. Write quickly to ward off your inner critic.
3. Speak from your heart.

Day Four and Beyond

As you reach the final day of your Anti-Bloat Jumpstart, I know what you'll be feeling. You'll feel lighter, stronger, more confident, and more self-centered (in a good way) than you've ever felt before. That's exactly the right mind-set for forging ahead and beginning the next phase of the *Flat Belly Diet:* the 28-day program that will give you the tools to manage your health and maintain your desired goal weight for the rest of your life.

THE FOUR-DAY ANTI-BLOAT MENU, DAY 1

DATE:

BREAKFAST

- ❏ 1 cup unsweetened cornflakes
- ❏ 1 cup skim milk
- ❏ ½ cup unsweetened applesauce
- ❏ ¼ cup roasted or raw unsalted sunflower seeds
- ❏ Glass of Sassy Water

MIND TRICK: Say hello, sunshine! Enjoy breakfast near a sunny window. Morning sunlight has been shown to be a mood booster and will set your body's master clock for maximum all-day energy.

LUNCH

- ❏ 4 oz organic deli turkey, rolled up
- ❏ 1 low-fat string cheese
- ❏ 1 pint fresh grape tomatoes
- ❏ Glass of Sassy Water

MIND TRICK: Put some color in your day. Before sitting down, arrange a few cut flowers in a vase and place it on the table. You're working hard on this diet. You deserve something special for your efforts.

SNACK

- ❏ Blueberry Smoothie: Blend 1 cup skim milk and 1 cup frozen unsweetened blueberries in blender for 1 minute. Transfer to glass and stir in 1 Tbsp cold-pressed organic flaxseed oil, or serve with 1 Tbsp sunflower or pumpkin seeds.

MIND TRICK: Take a virtual vacation. Put on some Hawaiian music while you're preparing your meal and transport yourself to a beach with lapping water and coconut palms. For good measure rub a little suntan oil on your face and inhale deeply. It's snowing outside? Nah. You're in Hawaii.

DINNER

- ❏ 1 cup cooked green beans
- ❏ 4 oz grilled tilapia
- ❏ ½ cup roasted red potatoes drizzled with 1 tsp olive oil
- ❏ Glass of Sassy Water

MIND TRICK: Resize your settings. Set your table with smaller plates and bowls. It'll make you feel like you have more food than you actually do.

JOURNAL, DAY 1

DATE: _____

BREAKFAST

MOOD: _____

THOUGHTS/CHALLENGES: _____

HUNGER BEFORE: -5 -3 0 3 5 7 | HUNGER AFTER: -5 -3 0 3 5 7

LUNCH

MOOD: _____

THOUGHTS/CHALLENGES: _____

HUNGER BEFORE: -5 -3 0 3 5 7 | HUNGER AFTER: -5 -3 0 3 5 7

SNACK

MOOD: _____

THOUGHTS/CHALLENGES: _____

HUNGER BEFORE: -5 -3 0 3 5 7 | HUNGER AFTER: -5 -3 0 3 5 7

DINNER

MOOD: _____

THOUGHTS/CHALLENGES: _____

HUNGER BEFORE: -5 -3 0 3 5 7 | HUNGER AFTER: -5 -3 0 3 5 7

Hunger Rating

−5 = STARVING. You want to devour the first thing you see and have a hard time slowing down.

−3 = OVERLY HUNGRY AND IRRITABLE. You feel like you waited too long to eat.

0 = MILD TO MODERATE HUNGER. You may have physical symptoms of hunger, like a growling tummy and that "I need to eat soon" feeling, but you aren't starving or experiencing any unpleasant symptoms such as a headache or shaking.

3 = HUNGER BUT NOT CRAVING FREE. You're full, but you don't feel quite satisfied; your thoughts are still focused on food.

5 = JUST RIGHT. Your hunger is gone, and you feel satisfied. Your mind is off food, and you're ready to take on the next task. You feel energized.

7 = A LITTLE TOO MUCH. You think you overdid it. Your tummy feels stretched and uncomfortable. You feel kind of sluggish.

THE FOUR-DAY ANTI-BLOAT MENU, DAY 2

DATE:

BREAKFAST

- ❏ 1 cup Rice Krispies®
- ❏ 1 cup skim milk
- ❏ ¼ cup roasted or raw unsalted sunflower seeds
- ❏ 4 oz pineapple tidbits canned in juice
- ❏ Glass of Sassy Water

MIND TRICK: Find a one-meal-only mantra. Pick a calming word or phrase, such as "I'm doing this diet for me." Repeat it after every bite.

LUNCH

- ❏ 3 oz chunk light tuna in water
- ❏ 1 cup steamed baby carrots
- ❏ 1 low-fat string cheese
- ❏ Glass of Sassy Water

MIND TRICK: Convert a friend. Invite a pal to have lunch with you today and explain your meal. Try to remember as many principles of the Jumpstart as possible. This will help you remember why you're doing this, even though it's such a departure from your normal routine.

SNACK

- ❏ Pineapple Smoothie: Blend 1 cup skim milk, 4 oz canned pineapple tidbits in juice, and a handful of ice in blender for 1 minute. Transfer to glass and stir in 1 Tbsp cold-pressed organic flaxseed oil, or serve with 1 Tbsp sunflower or pumpkin seeds.

MIND TRICK: Hang up some inspiration. Keep, say, your "skinny jeans" on a hanger in full view, so you pass them every day. They'll serve as a reminder of your ultimate weight loss goal. They *will* fit you again.

DINNER

- ❏ 1 cup fresh cremini mushrooms sautéed with 1 tsp olive oil
- ❏ 3 oz grilled chicken breast
- ❏ ½ cup cooked brown rice
- ❏ Glass of Sassy Water

MIND TRICK: Sing while you prepare dinner. According to German researchers, you can enjoy up to a 240 percent immunity boost as well as an increase of anti-stress hormones simply by singing.

JOURNAL, DAY 2

DATE:

BREAKFAST	
MOOD:	THOUGHTS/CHALLENGES:

HUNGER BEFORE: -5 -3 0 3 5 7   HUNGER AFTER: -5 -3 0 3 5 7

LUNCH	
MOOD:	THOUGHTS/CHALLENGES:

HUNGER BEFORE: -5 -3 0 3 5 7   HUNGER AFTER: -5 -3 0 3 5 7

SNACK	
MOOD:	THOUGHTS/CHALLENGES:

HUNGER BEFORE: -5 -3 0 3 5 7   HUNGER AFTER: -5 -3 0 3 5 7

DINNER	
MOOD:	THOUGHTS/CHALLENGES:

HUNGER BEFORE: -5 -3 0 3 5 7   HUNGER AFTER: -5 -3 0 3 5 7

Hunger Rating

–5 = STARVING. You want to devour the first thing you see and have a hard time slowing down.

–3 = OVERLY HUNGRY AND IRRITABLE. You feel like you waited too long to eat.

0 = MILD TO MODERATE HUNGER. You may have physical symptoms of hunger, like a growling tummy and that "I need to eat soon" feeling, but you aren't starving or experiencing any unpleasant symptoms such as a headache or shaking.

3 = HUNGER BUT NOT CRAVING FREE. You're full, but you don't feel quite satisfied; your thoughts are still focused on food.

5 = JUST RIGHT. Your hunger is gone, and you feel satisfied. Your mind is off food, and you're ready to take on the next task. You feel energized.

7 = A LITTLE TOO MUCH. You think you overdid it. Your tummy feels stretched and uncomfortable. You feel kind of sluggish.

THE FOUR-DAY ANTI-BLOAT MENU, DAY 3

DATE:

BREAKFAST

- ❏ 1 cup unsweetened cornflakes
- ❏ 1 cup skim milk
- ❏ ¼ cup roasted or raw unsalted sunflower seeds
- ❏ 2 Tbsp raisins
- ❏ Glass of Sassy Water

MIND TRICK: Focus on your moment. This morning, eat your breakfast with no distraction—no radio, no morning show, no newspaper. Focus on the flavor of each bite.

LUNCH

- ❏ 4 oz organic deli turkey, rolled up
- ❏ 1 low-fat string cheese
- ❏ 1 pint grape tomatoes
- ❏ Glass of Sassy Water

MIND TRICK: Bring in some bling. Serve your Sassy Water in the finest crystal glass you own. Make this your Flat Belly glass, and use it at every meal.

SNACK

- ❏ Peach Smoothie: Blend 1 cup skim milk and 1 cup frozen, unsweetened peaches in blender for 1 minute. Transfer to glass and stir in 1 Tbsp cold-pressed organic flaxseed oil, or serve with 1 Tbsp sunflower or pumpkin seeds.

MIND TRICK: Give thanks. Take a moment of gratitude for the food you are eating, the body you are nurturing, and the life you're enhancing. No need to get religious—it's perfectly okay to thank the peach farmer and your parents!

DINNER

- ❏ 1 cup cooked green beans
- ❏ 3 oz grilled or baked turkey breast cutlet
- ❏ ½ cup roasted red potatoes drizzled with 1 tsp olive oil
- ❏ Glass of Sassy Water

MIND TRICK: Think about yourself. Remember the list you compiled in Chapter 4, the one listing all the important people in your life? As you eat this meal, reflect on all you're doing to care for your body and your spirit.

JOURNAL, DAY 3

DATE: _____

BREAKFAST	
MOOD:	THOUGHTS/CHALLENGES:

HUNGER BEFORE: -5 -3 0 3 5 7   HUNGER AFTER: -5 -3 0 3 5 7

LUNCH	
MOOD:	THOUGHTS/CHALLENGES:

HUNGER BEFORE: -5 -3 0 3 5 7   HUNGER AFTER: -5 -3 0 3 5 7

SNACK	
MOOD:	THOUGHTS/CHALLENGES:

HUNGER BEFORE: -5 -3 0 3 5 7   HUNGER AFTER: -5 -3 0 3 5 7

DINNER	
MOOD:	THOUGHTS/CHALLENGES:

HUNGER BEFORE: -5 -3 0 3 5 7   HUNGER AFTER: -5 -3 0 3 5 7

Hunger Rating

−5 = STARVING. You want to devour the first thing you see and have a hard time slowing down.

−3 = OVERLY HUNGRY AND IRRITABLE. You feel like you waited too long to eat.

0 = MILD TO MODERATE HUNGER. You may have physical symptoms of hunger, like a growling tummy and that "I need to eat soon" feeling, but you aren't starving or experiencing any unpleasant symptoms such as a headache or shaking.

3 = HUNGER BUT NOT CRAVING FREE. You're full, but you don't feel quite satisfied; your thoughts are still focused on food.

5 = JUST RIGHT. Your hunger is gone, and you feel satisfied. Your mind is off food, and you're ready to take on the next task. You feel energized.

7 = A LITTLE TOO MUCH. You think you overdid it. Your tummy feels stretched and uncomfortable. You feel kind of sluggish.

THE FOUR-DAY ANTI-BLOAT MENU, DAY 4

DATE:

BREAKFAST	
❏ 1 packet instant Cream of Wheat®	**MIND TRICK:** Laugh it up. A 4-year-old laughs around 400 times a day; an adult, around 15. Today, even if you're alone when you sit down to your meal, laugh at your bowl of Cream of Wheat, howl at your glass of Sassy Water.
❏ 1 cup skim milk	
❏ ¼ cup roasted or raw unsalted sunflower seeds	
❏ 2 dried plums	
❏ Glass of Sassy Water	

LUNCH	
❏ 4 oz organic deli turkey, rolled up	**MIND TRICK:** Arrange your plate. Take a few minutes to prepare today's lunch with the flair of a gourmet chef. Wrap the turkey slices around the cheese and carrots, then slice on the bias and arrange. Garnish with a few sprigs of fresh herbs.
❏ 1 cup steamed baby carrots	
❏ 1 low-fat string cheese	
❏ Glass of Sassy Water	

SNACK	
❏ Strawberry Smoothie: Blend 1 cup skim milk and 1 cup frozen, unsweetened strawberries in blender for 1 minute. Transfer to glass and stir in 1 Tbsp cold-pressed organic flaxseed oil, or serve with 1 Tbsp sunflower or pumpkin seeds.	**MIND TRICK:** Before you sit down to eat, close your eyes and say something kind and reassuring about your body. Mention how much you love your arms or how people tell you you have great eyes or a fantastic smile.

DINNER	
❏ 1 cup yellow squash sautéed with 1 tsp olive oil	**MIND TRICK:** Serve today's dinner on your best china. Set a proper place setting with the good silver and the damask napkins.
❏ 3 oz grilled chicken breast	
❏ ½ cup cooked brown rice	
❏ Glass of Sassy Water	

JOURNAL, DAY 4

DATE: _____

BREAKFAST	
MOOD:	THOUGHTS/CHALLENGES:

HUNGER BEFORE: -5 -3 0 3 5 7 | HUNGER AFTER: -5 -3 0 3 5 7

LUNCH	
MOOD:	THOUGHTS/CHALLENGES:

HUNGER BEFORE: -5 -3 0 3 5 7 | HUNGER AFTER: -5 -3 0 3 5 7

SNACK	
MOOD:	THOUGHTS/CHALLENGES:

HUNGER BEFORE: -5 -3 0 3 5 7 | HUNGER AFTER: -5 -3 0 3 5 7

DINNER	
MOOD:	THOUGHTS/CHALLENGES:

HUNGER BEFORE: -5 -3 0 3 5 7 | HUNGER AFTER: -5 -3 0 3 5 7

Hunger Rating

−5 = STARVING. You want to devour the first thing you see and have a hard time slowing down.

−3 = OVERLY HUNGRY AND IRRITABLE. You feel like you waited too long to eat.

0 = MILD TO MODERATE HUNGER. You may have physical symptoms of hunger, like a growling tummy and that "I need to eat soon" feeling, but you aren't starving or experiencing any unpleasant symptoms such as a headache or shaking.

3 = HUNGER BUT NOT CRAVING FREE. You're full, but you don't feel quite satisfied; your thoughts are still focused on food.

5 = JUST RIGHT. Your hunger is gone, and you feel satisfied. Your mind is off food, and you're ready to take on the next task. You feel energized.

7 = A LITTLE TOO MUCH. You think you overdid it. Your tummy feels stretched and uncomfortable. You feel kind of sluggish.

READ A FLAT BELLY
SUCCESS
STORY

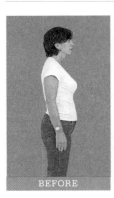

BEFORE

Colleen O'Neill-Groves

AGE: 45

POUNDS LOST:

6

IN 32 DAYS

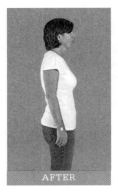

AFTER

ALL-OVER INCHES LOST:

5.5

I'VE SPENT MY WHOLE LIFE ON ONE DIET OR ANOTHER," LAMENTS Colleen O'Neill-Groves. "I really tried them all—A to Z—none with much lasting success. There was always a downside somewhere." She goes on to explain that on all of the diets, when she *did* lose weight, the first place she lost fat was in her face and her breasts, both of which looked okay to begin with. And her belly—which needed the fat loss the *most*—was always the last place to give it up. Another aspect she couldn't get past was that she was always, always hungry. "I would finish lunch and start wondering, *Okay, how soon can I have my snack?*"

The *Flat Belly Diet,* says the 45-year-old mother of three, is all things great and good. She calls the food amazing but explains that for the plan to work, you have to rid yourself of any preconceived notions about things like olive oil and nuts. She kept wondering how anyone could possibly lose weight on all the scrumptious food. "The bars were overall a pleasant surprise. And the waffle, pesto sauce, pizza . . . just great stuff. Sure, on these other diets I had unlimited veggies—but after a while, you can't look at another lettuce leaf. And you never got wraps or avocado or pesto sauce."

Colleen says on this diet, you know exactly what you're taking in and the value it represents for your body. It made her realize how much junk she was eating in a given day and how many calories she stuffed herself with without a second thought. "I'm very aware of my body because I exercise so much," she says, "so if there's ever an opportunity out there to take better care of myself, I'm going to take it."

It wasn't all nirvana, though, admits Colleen. She describes the first 4 days—the Anti-Bloat Jumpstart—as "not that easy," but adds that it was only 4 days and "in the end, it was definitely a perfect way to start off. I figured I could do anything for 4 days. Now, when I celebrate a bit too much over a weekend, I actually put myself *back* on the jumpstart diet to make up for it."

In the first 4 weeks, Colleen lost 6 pounds. "I'm not that big to begin with," she says, "so I was really happy with my results. I lost an inch on each thigh, an inch around each arm, and a few in my belly—while my breast size remained the same—which is exactly what I had hoped for."

THE FLAT BELLY
DIET
RULES

WOW. Isn't it amazing how dramatically you can change the way you think and feel in only 4 short days? You've just completed a major milestone on the *Flat Belly Diet*—you've mastered the elusive art of banishing bloat from your life forever. And, if you completed each Mind Trick, you've accumulated lots of little useful strategies you can employ anywhere, anytime, to boost your confidence and stay motivated. But now that you've seen how a flatter belly looks and felt the renewed confidence that comes from experiencing such fast results, you're ready to move on to the next—and most life-changing—phase of the *Flat Belly Diet:* You're ready to lose belly fat.

For just about everyone who's ever tried to lose weight, the word *diet* means long lists of forbidden foods, nonstop hunger, willpower struggles, and, eventually, a return to "normal" eating once you've met your goal. For Cynthia and me, *diet* has an altogether different meaning, one that's inspired by the National Institutes of Health, which simply defines diet as "what a person eats and drinks; a type of eating plan." The *Flat Belly Diet* is a way of eating, one that allows you to get to, and then stay at, your ideal weight, while optimizing your health and energy and slashing your odds of getting nearly every chronic disease.

Our plan, as you know, makes a specific promise: less belly fat. And less belly fat will, in turn, reduce your risk of disease. But even after we'd found the research supporting the notion that a particular food group—those beloved MUFAs—could accomplish that, and even after Cynthia worked out the calorie counts and made sure that the nutrient requirements of the average woman could be met, we still had a bit of work to do. I knew that the *Flat Belly Diet* was going to have to compete with a whole shelf (or many shelves) full of popular plans, every one of them promising significant weight loss. I knew that to stand out on that shelf, it had to offer something—or many things—that other diets don't have.

Step one was asking *Prevention* readers what they loved and hated about traditional weight-loss diets. I quickly found that one woman's dietary nightmare is another's dream, which is probably why there's a diet book for every woman out there these days. Books exist for people with certain blood types, people who hate carbs, people with fat phobias, people who like, um, cabbage soup—whoever those unique and adventurous individuals might be. But I talked with Cynthia and learned a few universal truths about diets that actually work for the vast majority of people.

- They offer sound advice and deliver on their promises. (Check. I would offer *Prevention* readers nothing less.)
- They offer a plan that women can return to again and again, whenever their favorite jeans feel a little too snug. (Check. The Four-Day Anti-Bloat Jump-

DID YOU KNOW **?**

A 1-pound fat loss is something to celebrate—though not, of course, with a fattening treat! One pound of fat is the equivalent of 4 sticks of butter. Close your eyes and imagine 4 sticks of butter gone from your belly. This is what you can do for yourself!

start is an effective, safe solution you can turn to whenever you need an instant svelting.)

■ They are easy to live with. (Check . . . ?)

Ahhh, that was the rub: How could we devise a plan that worked for everybody all the time? I thought about this a long while and worried that it wasn't possible simply because there are as many definitions of "perfect" as there are readers of this book. Cynthia assured me, however, that it *was* possible! Her years of counseling dieters—and her rigorous planning for the *Flat Belly Diet*—are the backbone of this lifestyle. It was possible because the *Flat Belly Diet* offers:

■ FOCUS ON HEALTH AND ENERGY. Anyone can lose weight on a 1,200-calorie diet. But here's what you'll also lose: muscle, bone density, zest for living, sanity, and, if you follow a diet like that for too long, your sense of humor. (I've seen it happen!) Featuring satisfying, wholesome foods and a 1,600-calorie-a-day guideline, the *Flat Belly Diet* is as healthy as they come.

■ FLAVOR. It's food, after all! We consider no diet "complete" or "healthy" unless it's filled with delicious foods and meals any palate can enjoy. This plan offers as much taste as nutrition.

■ REALITY. We wouldn't ask anyone to do something that we weren't willing—or able—to do ourselves.

■ FLEXIBILITY. If you're pressed for time, we wanted you to be able to assemble meals quickly, with little or no cooking. If, on the other hand, you want to cook for your family or friends, we wanted to make that easy without endangering your goal. And finally, if you don't like a suggested meal, you should be able to swap it out for something you *do* want to eat. The *Flat Belly Diet* is about as flexible as it gets.

Three Rules to Eat By

OVER THE NEXT 28 days—and beyond—you are going to eat very well. How does Spicy Shrimp with Chili Bean Glaze sound? Chicago-Style Hot Dog, anyone? How about a Chocolate Chip Cherry Waffle? They're just a few of the anti-"diet" dishes you'll be eating. And it won't be a lot of work. We've developed two different ways to follow the *Flat Belly Diet:* The first, in Chapter 7, is perfect if you're too busy to even think about cooking dinner. It's also a great way to familiarize yourself with this new way of eating, because it lays everything out for you. You don't have to think about portion size because everything is preportioned. Chapter 8 is loaded with MUFA-packed recipes and meal additions that will allow you to follow the *Flat Belly Diet* when convenience foods may not be an option—family dinner night, for example, or when you're entertaining. Both plans adhere to three very important *Flat Belly Diet* rules that you must follow if you expect to reap the health and weight-loss rewards on this plan. They are:

▨ Rule #1: Stick to 400 calories per meal.

▨ Rule #2: Never go more than 4 hours without eating.

▨ Rule #3: Eat a MUFA at every meal.

RULE #1: STICK TO 400 CALORIES PER MEAL.

YOU'VE PROBABLY NOTICED from looking at the list of MUFAs on page 37 that they're not exactly low-cal choices. They're all foods—nuts, oils, chocolate—that you're usually told to avoid when you're trying to lose weight. But because these

MUFAs are so essential to losing belly fat, calorie control in what surrounds them takes on extra importance. All the meals in the *Flat Belly Diet* provide a MUFA *and* total about 400 calories. An added bonus of this controlled-calorie plan is that you can substitute one whole meal for another. You can eat breakfast for dinner or lunch for breakfast. If you like, you can even eat four breakfast meals in one day. That's part of the ease of this plan. I don't expect that you'll love every single meal. But on the other hand, if you find a few you absolutely adore, it's perfectly okay to enjoy them to your heart's content.

This diet is 1,600 calories per day because that's how much it takes for a woman of average height, frame size, and activity level to get to and stay at her ideal body weight (men who want customized calorie counts can go to **flatbellydiet.com**). So 1,600 calories is not a starvation plan—it's enough to keep up your energy, support your immune system, and maintain your precious calorie-burning muscle. That means you won't feel run-down, cranky, irritable, moody, or hungry. But you also won't be eating enough calories to hang on to your belly.

RULE #2: NEVER GO MORE THAN 4 HOURS WITHOUT EATING.

I DON'T HAVE to tell you that a diet won't work if it makes you feel hungry or tired. That's why on the *Flat Belly Diet*, you're *required* to eat every 4 hours. Waiting too long to eat can cause you to become so hungry (and irritable) that it's hard to even think clearly. That means you won't have the energy or patience to think through the healthiest meal choice, let alone prepare one. You'll probably want to tear into the first thing you see (bag of chips, handfuls of dry cereal straight from the box, cookies, and so on), and you'll probably have a hard time slowing down while you eat and not reaching for seconds.

Snacks are especially important, but when you eat them is entirely up to you. I like to have a snack in the evening while I'm reading manuscripts, but some of the editors I work with need a small meal in the afternoon to keep them going until dinnertime. Your snacktime is entirely personal and entirely essential. To help you include your snack every day, Cynthia has created a variety of Snack Packs that you can prepare ahead of time and take with you each morning. They're portable and MUFA-loaded. Use the Snack Pack as a floating meal.

RULE #3: EAT A MUFA AT EVERY MEAL.

"A MUFA AT every meal" has almost become a mantra for me. As you know, "MUFA" (MOO-fah) stands for "monounsaturated fatty acid," a type of heart-healthy, disease-fighting, "good" fat found in foods like almonds, peanut butter, olive oil, avocados, even chocolate. MUFAs are an *un*saturated fat and have the exact opposite effect of the unhealthy saturated and trans fats you've heard about in the news.

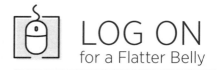

LOG ON
for a Flatter Belly

At **www.flatbellydiet.com,** women and men of all shapes and sizes can find everything they need to faithfully follow the entire *Flat Belly Diet* program for life. There, you can:

▓ Create your very own menu plans from hundreds of delicious MUFA-packed, calorie-controlled meals.

▓ Track your nutritional intake.

▓ Generate personal shopping lists.

▓ Read more about our success stories, whose profiles you see throughout this book, or nominate your own!

▓ Customize the Anti-Bloat Jumpstart and *Flat Belly Diet* if you are a vegetarian or have other dietary needs.

But there's more! MUFAs are delicious in and of themselves. Who doesn't love drizzling olive oil over a salad or grabbing a handful of chocolate chips? You'll find the MUFA-rich foods incorporated into the meal plans and Snack Packs. You can substitute one MUFA for another as long as the calorie counts are nearly equivalent. For example, you can exchange almond butter (200 calories) for semisweet chocolate chips (207). For precise MUFA serving amounts per meal, consult the chart on the opposite page. Better yet, copy this chart and post it on the inside door of your pantry. To get better acquainted with the five MUFA groups and learn how to buy, store, and prepare them, turn to page 103.

YOUR MUFA SERVING CHART

FOOD	SERVING	CALORIES
SOYBEANS (EDAMAME), SHELLED AND BOILED	1 cup	298
SEMISWEET CHOCOLATE CHIPS	1/4 cup	207
ALMOND BUTTER	2 Tbsp	200
CASHEW BUTTER	2 Tbsp	190
SUNFLOWER SEED BUTTER	2 Tbsp	190
NATURAL PEANUT BUTTER, CRUNCHY	2 Tbsp	188
NATURAL PEANUT BUTTER, SMOOTH	2 Tbsp	188
TAHINI (SESAME SEED PASTE)	2 Tbsp	178
PUMPKIN SEEDS	2 Tbsp	148
CANOLA OIL	1 Tbsp	124
FLAXSEED OIL (COLD-PRESSED ORGANIC)	1 Tbsp	120
MACADAMIA NUTS	2 Tbsp	120
SAFFLOWER OIL (HIGH OLEIC)	1 Tbsp	120
SESAME OR SOYBEAN OIL	1 Tbsp	120
SUNFLOWER OIL (HIGH OLEIC)	1 Tbsp	120
WALNUT OIL	1 Tbsp	120
OLIVE OIL	1 Tbsp	119
PEANUT OIL	1 Tbsp	119
PINE NUTS	2 Tbsp	113
BRAZIL NUTS	2 Tbsp	110
HAZELNUTS	2 Tbsp	110
PEANUTS	2 Tbsp	110
ALMONDS	2 Tbsp	109
CASHEWS	2 Tbsp	100
AVOCADO, CALIFORNIA (HASS)	1/4 cup	96
PECANS	2 Tbsp	90
SUNFLOWER SEEDS	2 Tbsp	90
BLACK OLIVE TAPENADE	2 Tbsp	88
PISTACHIOS	2 Tbsp	88
WALNUTS	2 Tbsp	82
PESTO SAUCE	1 Tbsp	80
AVOCADO, FLORIDA	1/4 cup	69
GREEN OLIVE TAPENADE	2 Tbsp	54
GREEN OR BLACK OLIVES	10 large	50

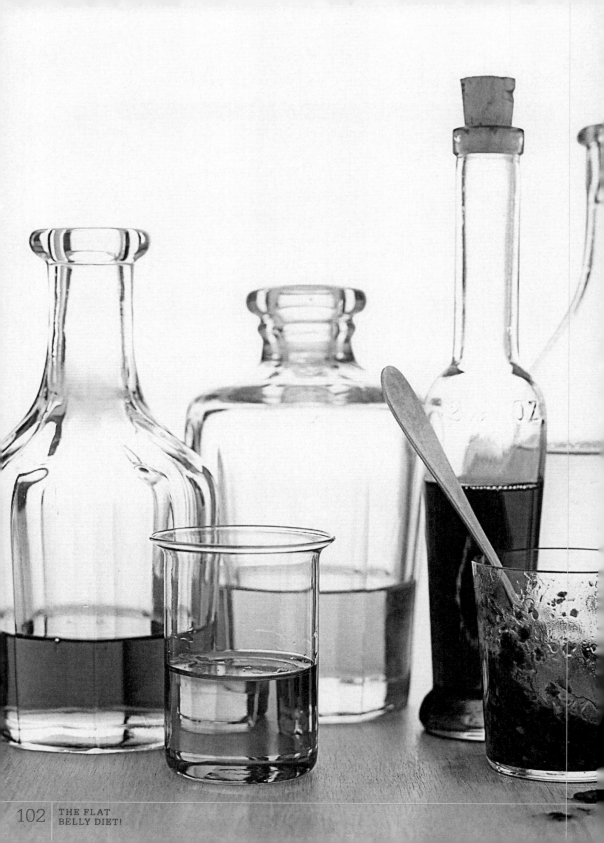

THE FLAT
BELLY DIET!

1. Oils

ANOINT YOUR MEALS with the most versatile MUFAs in the kitchen. Choose your oil based on use—cooking or drizzling—and flavor—strong or mild.

HOW TO BUY AND USE: We recommend expeller pressed oils, a chemical-free extraction process. This natural method allows the oil to retain its natural color, aroma, and nutrients. Cold-pressed oil is expeller pressed in a heat-controlled environment to keep temperatures below 120°F. This is important for delicate oils like flaxseed.

HOW TO STORE: Choose a container that holds only what you'll use within 2 months. As each container empties, it fills with oxygen, which causes the oil to oxidize, or deteriorate. This eventually creates a stale or bitter taste (like wet cardboard) and contributes to a breakdown of vitamin E and those precious MUFAs. Opt for dark glass jars or tins (rather than clear plastic bottles) to protect the oil from light, another source of flavor-sapping oxidation. You can store opened bottles of olive, canola, and peanut oils in a dark, cool place, such as the back of your pantry, but flaxseed oil should always be kept in the refrigerator because it breaks down more quickly at warmer temperatures.

HISTORY

Oils extracted from plant foods have been used in nearly every culture around the globe since ancient times. A 4,000-year-old kitchen unearthed by an archaeologist in Indiana revealed that large slabs of rock had been used to crush nuts, then extract the oil.

FUN FACT!

SAFFLOWER OIL LABELED "HIGH-OLEIC" CONTAINS THE MOST BENEFICIAL MUFAS, FOLLOWED BY OLIVE OIL, AND THEN CANOLA OIL.

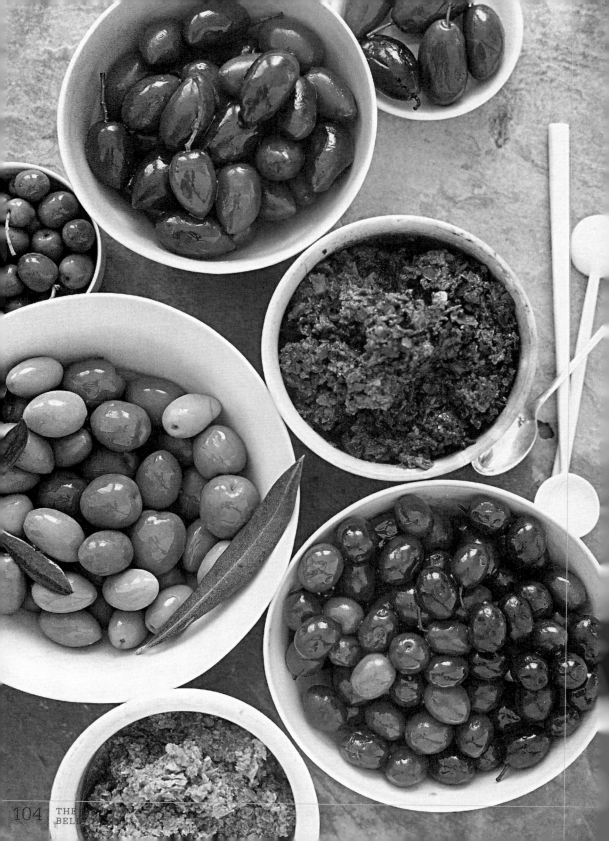

2. Olives

THERE'S AN OLIVE out there just for you. Choose your color (black or green) and pick your flavor (salty, sweet, or spicy). When you're all olived out, switch to tapenade, a deliciously pungent spread made from the crushed fruit.

HOW TO BUY AND USE: Fresh olives are available during the summer in specialty markets, but don't be lured unless you're a serious gourmet; they're incredibly bitter and inedible, thanks to a naturally occurring compound called oleuropin. Instead, choose the more appetizing olives at deli counters, which are sometimes pasteurized and cured in either oil, salt, or brine, and flavored with herbs or hot chilies. Olives can be purchased in jars and cans, as well as in bulk.

HOW TO STORE: Olives should be stored in the refrigerator after opening, either in the jar or an airtight container. If you bought your olives in cans, transfer any leftover into another airtight container before storing in the fridge.

HISTORY

Native to coastal regions of the Mediterranean, Asia, and areas of Africa, olives have been cultivated since 6000 BC and are one of the oldest known foods. These gems were brought to America by Spanish and Portuguese explorers during the 15th and 16th centuries and to California missions in the late 18th century. Today, most commercial olives are grown in Spain, Italy, Greece, and Turkey.

FUN FACT! TRADITIONAL CHINESE MEDICINE USES OLIVE SOUP AS A SORE-THROAT RECIPE—THE ONLY OCCURRENCE OF THE OLIVE IN CHINESE CUISINE.

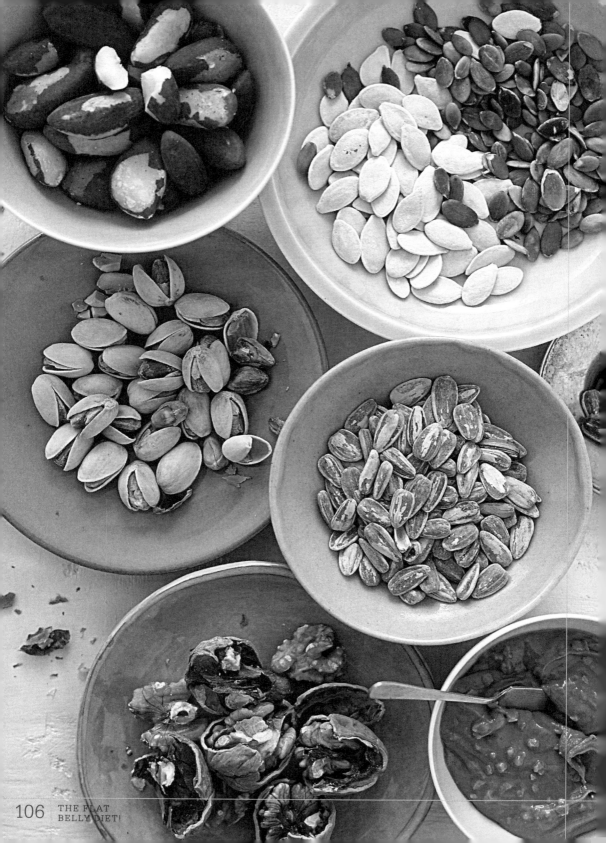

3. Nuts and Seeds

THESE MUFAS HAVE long been revered for their high levels of protein, fiber, and antioxidants (not to mention those healthy fats!). Sprinkle on yogurt, cereal, and salads; use as a topping for fish and chicken; or just snack on them out of hand.

HOW TO BUY AND USE: Nuts and seeds are sold in a variety of ways, including vacuum-sealed cans, glass jars, sealed bags, and in bulk. They can be whole, sliced, or chopped; raw or roasted; in or out of the shell. If purchasing in bulk, select a market that has high turnover and uses covered bins so they'll be perfectly fresh. Unshelled nuts should be free from cracks or holes, feel somewhat heavy for their size, and not rattle in the shell. Shelled nuts should be plump and look uniform in size and shape.

HOW TO STORE: Due to their high fat content, nuts and seeds tend to go rancid quickly once their shells are removed, especially if they're exposed to heat, light, and humidity during storage, so buy them as fresh as possible. When kept in a cool, dry place in an airtight container, raw, unshelled nuts will keep from 6 months to a year, while shelled nuts will stay fresh for 3 to 4 months under the same conditions. Shelled nuts can be stored for 4 months in a refrigerator and 6 months in a freezer.

HISTORY

Nuts and seeds have a long, extensive history. Almonds were prized by Egypt's pharaohs. The use of flaxseed goes as far back as the Stone Age and ancient Greece. Native Americans have been using sunflower seeds for more than 5,000 years, and peanuts were a staple of the Aztec diet.

FUN FACT !

MACADAMIA NUTS PROVIDE MORE MUFA THAN ANY OTHER NUT OR SEED.

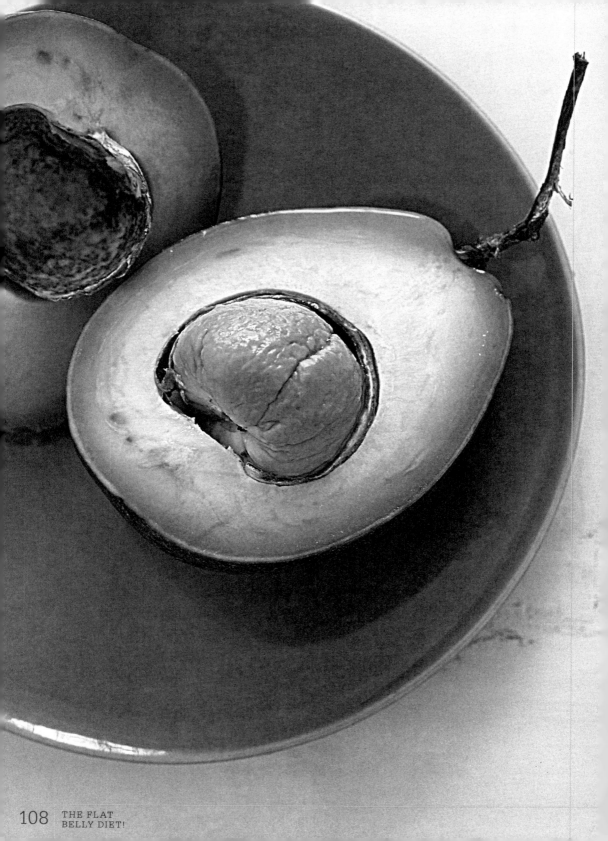

4. Avocados

ONCE A LUXURY FOOD reserved for royalty, supercreamy avocado is a feast of riches. Delicious mashed into a dip or sliced onto a salad, this MUFA is like butter, only better.

HOW TO BUY AND USE: When selecting any avocado, look for a fruit with slightly soft skin that yields slightly when you press it with your thumb. Avoid bruised, cracked, or indented fruit. Those with teardrop-shaped necks have usually been tree ripened and will have a richer taste than rounded specimens. Once it's ripe, use a sharp knife to slice it lengthwise, guiding the knife gently around the pit. Then twist the two halves against each other in opposite directions to separate. The pit will still be lodged in one half. Carefully nudge the knife into the pit and twist it out to discard. You can either gently peel away the skin or carefully score the avocado while still in the peel, cutting into long slices or chunks, and use a spoon to separate it from the skin.

HOW TO STORE: A whole, ripe avocado with the skin on will keep in the refrigerator for a day or two. A slightly unripe avocado can be ripened in just a day or two by storing it in a paper bag and keeping it on the counter. To prevent a leftover portion from browning, coat the exposed flesh with lemon juice, wrap tightly in plastic wrap, and store in the refrigerator.

HISTORY

Avocados have been cultivated in South and Central America since 8000 BC. They were not introduced to the United States until the early 20th century, when they were first planted in California and Florida.

FUN FACT !

HASS AVOCADOS HAVE A MUCH CREAMIER CONSISTENCY THAN THEIR FLORIDA COUNTERPARTS AND PROVIDE ALMOST TWICE THE MUFA PER QUARTER-CUP SERVING.

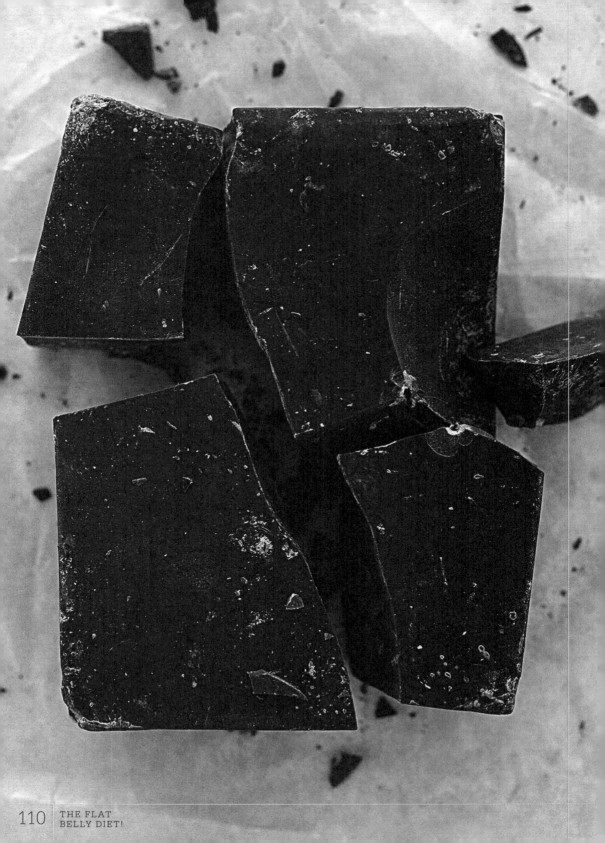

5. Dark Chocolate

OUR MOST BELOVED MUFA. The one that makes us swoon. The one that makes every meal or snack a little bit sweeter. And the one that makes everyone want to start the *Flat Belly Diet*—and never stop.

HOW TO BUY AND USE: Semisweet and other dark chocolates are low enough in sugar and high enough in monounsaturated fats to get the MUFA accolade in our book. Chocolates with a higher "cacao," or cocoa, content—the package usually lists the percentage—are typically darker, less sweet, and slightly more bitter, but in a good way. If you're used to milk chocolate, go dark gradually so you train your tastebuds to appreciate the stronger flavor of real, dark chocolate. You can buy chocolate in large chunks (popular with the baking set), as molded bars, or in chip form. I like chips because they're so easy to measure and use. (And when I want chocolate, I don't want to hassle with a knife and a grater!)

HOW TO STORE: Keep dark chocolate that's in its original sealed package in a cool dry area (60 to 75°F). Once opened, chocolate should be transferred to an airtight container or bag and stashed in the fridge (good) or freezer (best). During prolonged storage, chocolate will often "bloom," or develop a white blush. It's perfectly safe to eat, though not very appetizing to look at. One solution: Melt it—the bloom will disappear.

HISTORY

You're not the only one who loves chocolate. The ancient Mayans and Aztecs touted it as a food of the gods—and it's been a culinary mainstay ever since.

FUN FACT !

CHOCOLATE REALLY DOES MELT IN YOUR MOUTH BECAUSE ITS MELTING POINT IS SLIGHTLY BELOW HUMAN BODY TEMPERATURE.

READ A FLAT BELLY
SUCCESS
STORY

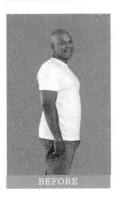

BEFORE

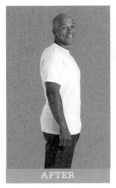

AFTER

Kevin Martin

AGE: 50

POUNDS LOST:

13.5

IN 32 DAYS

ALL-OVER INCHES LOST:

11.5

" IT'S NOT LIKE I DIDN'T CONTRIB-UTE TO THIS BELLY," LAMENTS Kevin Martin. "I'm a supervisor. So I ride around all day in my truck. You know how that is. You spend your day eating lots and lots of stuff that's not good for you. I'd head out to work at 6 a.m., and I'd stop on the way and get my coffee, and I might get two dough-nuts to go with it. By nine, I'm getting a bacon, egg, and cheese sandwich and a Snapple. That's breakfast. By twelve, I'm eating pizza or a big huge sand-wich, and that holds me until two, when it's time for a couple of Funny Bones and a drink. At four, I get home and go straight for the cookies in the cabinet, and then it's dinnertime." After dinner, it's poker on the computer. The next day? "Same thing all over again." After a long pause, he asks: "Is it any wonder that spare tire around my waist was slowly inflating?

"I wanted to lose 12 to 15 pounds and get rid of that spare tire," says the 50-year-old, adding that he's never been on a diet before—not successfully, anyway. He tried them several times with his wife but never stayed on one more than a couple of days.

This time, he says, was different. "I guess the timing was just right with this one. Summer was coming. And I wanted to be able to take off my shirt in public." He also knew he needed something to get him off the computer—playing online poker had become his nightly activity—and into the gym. "I belonged to a gym but never went. I was paying all that money for nothing. So because I was also on the [Flat Belly] exercise program, I started going to the gym again."

Kevin admits that the first 4 days—the Anti-Bloat Jumpstart—were a challenge for him. Going cold turkey from coffee was hard enough, he recollects. But giving up all the junk food? That was *really* hard for him. Still, he was committed. And he stuck to it. What kept him going was his athlete's sensibility. "I wanted to finish it. Get to day 32. I knew I would, too. I used to be a jock, and I played all kinds of sports. When you're an athlete, you start something, you finish it."

After the first full week, he was amazed at how great he was beginning to feel. He's happy he's doing something productive for himself *and* his body. Now when he gets home from work, instead of going for the cookies and the computer, he heads for the gym or takes a ride on his bike—or sometimes both. He has the energy now, he says. "I feel a lot better. I'm not tired ever—or hungry. My main objective was to be able to take my shirt off in public, and I'm there. Now that I've lost all this weight, I realize how terribly I had been treating my body. I won't be doing *that* again," he says. "Ever."

THE FOUR-WEEK PLAN: QUICK-AND-EASY MEALS

UNLIKE MOST OTHER diets, the *Flat Belly Diet* doesn't require you to follow a day-by-day, meal-by-meal menu. Say it with me: Hallelujah! Instead, you will have a prescribed schedule of meals (four per day, including a Snack Pack) and a predetermined calorie count per meal and snack (roughly 400). Beyond that, we don't dictate what to eat when. Instead, we offer suggestions—and lots of them. *All of the meals are interchangeable*, so you can mix and match all you want. Our test panelists happily reported that this freedom of choice made it a breeze for them to follow the plan faithfully—even beyond the 4-week test period.

DID YOU KNOW **?**

Being overweight or obese can cause cancer, shows a new study by researchers at the University of Oxford. Scientists studied more than one million British women, looking at the relationship between body mass index and cancer. Obese and overweight women were twice as prone to developing endometrial cancer and cancer of the esophagus than women of normal weight. They also had a 53 percent greater risk of developing kidney cancer and a 24 percent greater risk of developing pancreatic cancer.[1]

Remember, you will eat four 400-calorie meals each day: three meals plus one Snack Pack. Meals are categorized here as breakfast, lunch, and dinner, but because every single one follows the *Flat Belly* "400 calories with a MUFA" rule, you can shuffle them however you like. If you want Pineapple-Ham Pizza for breakfast and Apple-Cinnamon Waffles for dinner, go for it! There are 28 meals to choose from in each category, so, if you like, you can go for maximum variety and have something different for every meal, every day, for 4 weeks. On the other hand, if you find one breakfast you love and want to make it part of your morning routine every day, that's fine, too. (Join the creature-of-habit club. I've eaten the same breakfast every day for 3 years!) For leisurely days when you have more time on your hands and feel like cooking, turn to Chapter 8, where you'll find more than 80 fabulous *Flat Belly Diet* recipes.

Wondering what you'll do when you don't even have time to slap together a sandwich? Have no fear: At the end of this chapter is a list of 61 Ready-Made Meals, including meal replacement bars, healthy frozen dinners, and even in-a-pinch fast-food options you can pair with a MUFA serving from the chart on page 101.

You may be tempted to create your own meals right off the bat, but we caution you against this, at least for the first 28 days. It's important for you to get into the rhythm of the *Flat Belly Diet* way of eating first. Once you are fully acquainted with the portion sizes, MUFA servings, and basic composition of the meals, feel free to create your own meals as often as you like. However, customizing the meals to your taste is easy. The two questions below will clarify the most important points for you to keep in mind when altering the meals in this chapter.

The Food Questions

Can I swap out ingredients in a meal?

Yes and no. You should not move items from one meal to another—that is, you can't delete your MUFA from breakfast and add it to lunch. But you *can* swap out foods within a meal, as long as:

▪ They're within the same food group, such as tomatoes and red peppers or turkey and chicken; and

▪ The food you added provides about the same number of calories as the food you took out. The calories for each ingredient appear in parentheses.

Do I have to buy these exact brands?

Cynthia selected particular brands because of their taste, quality, availability, and, most importantly, nutritional value. The nutritional quality of foods in certain categories varies widely, so she scoured the supermarket aisles, read countless labels, and hand-picked the high-quality brands that met her tough nutritional standards. Including these foods guarantee steady weight loss because their precise calorie level per serving has been incorporated into the plan. So, yes, I encourage you to use these brands. However, if you can't or prefer not to, simply replace them with comparable foods with as close to the same calorie levels.

Flat Belly Breakfasts

Among our testers—and their families!—the Cherry-Chocolate Waffle on the next page was a huge hit. MUFAs are in **boldface**, and ingredient calorie counts are in parentheses.

Apple-Almond Oatmeal: ½ cup dry Quaker® Old Fashioned Quick 1-Minute Oats (150) (cooked with water to consistency of your choice), mixed with 1 large apple, sliced (116), and sprinkled with apple pie spice and 2 Tbsp **almonds** (109)
■ **Total Calories = 375**

Apple-Cinnamon Waffle:
2 LifeStream® Organic FlaxPlus® frozen waffles, toasted (200), topped with 1 cup Mott's® Natural Style Unsweetened Apple Sauce (100) and sprinkled with cinnamon, nutmeg, and 2 Tbsp **walnuts** (82)
■ **Total Calories = 382**

Avocado-Tomato Herbed Breakfast Tacos: 4 6-inch corn tortillas, warmed (180), spread with 2 Laughing Cow® Light Garlic & Herb Wedges (70) and filled evenly with ½ cup Organic Valley® 100% Egg Whites scrambled with cooking spray (50) and 4 fresh basil leaves (0); sprinkle with 1 fresh sliced plum tomato (12) and ¼ cup sliced **avocado** (96)
■ **Total Calories = 408**

Banana-Pecan Oatmeal: ½ cup dry Quaker® Old Fashioned Quick 1-Minute Oats (cooked with water to consistency of your choice) (150) mixed with 1 cup sliced banana (140) and sprinkled with cinnamon, nutmeg, and 2 Tbsp **pecans** (90)
■ **Total Calories = 380**

Banana Split Oatmeal: ½ cup dry Quaker® Old Fashioned Quick 1-Minute Oats (cooked with water to consistency of your choice) (150) mixed with ¼ cup microwaved frozen strawberries (20) and topped with ¼ cup sliced banana (35), 1 Tbsp semisweet chocolate chips (50), and 2 Tbsp **peanuts** (110)
■ **Total Calories = 365**

Banana Waffle: 2 LifeStream® Organic FlaxPlus® frozen waffles, toasted (200), topped with ½ cup sliced banana (70) and sprinkled with cinnamon, nutmeg, and 2 Tbsp **pecans** (90)
■ **Total Calories = 360**

Blueberry Nut Oatmeal: ¾ cup dry Quaker® Old Fashioned Quick 1-Minute Oats (cooked with water to consistency of your choice) (225) mixed with 1 cup Cascadian Farm® organic frozen blueberries, warmed in microwave for 1 minute (70), and 2 Tbsp **cashews** (100)
■ **Total Calories = 395**

Breakfast BLT: 1 Thomas'® 100% Whole Wheat English Muffin (120) spread with 2 Tbsp **black olive tapenade** (88) and topped with ½ fresh plum tomato, sliced (6), 3 large romaine lettuce leaves (3), 2 slices Applegate Farms® cooked organic turkey bacon (60), and 1 slice Applegate Farms® Organic Muenster Käse Cheese (85)

▓ **Total Calories = 362**

Breakfast Tacos: 4 6-inch corn tortillas, warmed (180), filled evenly with 4 scrambled egg whites (½ cup Organic Valley® 100% Egg Whites makes about 1 cup scrambled eggs) (50), ½ cup fresh baby spinach leaves (3), ¼ cup salsa (40), and ¼ cup sliced **avocado** (96)

▓ **Total Calories = 369**

Cashew Crunch: 1 slice Food For Life® Ezekiel 4:9® Sesame Sprouted Bread, toasted (80), spread with 2 Tbsp **cashew butter** (190) and sprinkled with ¼ cup raisins (130)

▓ **Total Calories = 400**

Cherry-Chocolate Waffle:
1 LifeStream® Organic FlaxPlus® frozen waffle (100) topped with 1 cup frozen Cascadian Farm® Organic Pitted Dark Sweet Cherries, thawed (90), and sprinkled with nutmeg and ¼ cup **semisweet chocolate chips** (207)

▓ **Total Calories = 397**

SASS FROM SASS

"Why So Many Calorie Counts?"

The numbers in the parentheses correspond to the calorie content of each ingredient. I provide them for a few reasons: First, to help you become familiar with the calorie levels of various ingredients—you may be surprised to find out just how many or few calories there are in certain foods. The second reason is to help you customize the plan. If you dislike a certain ingredient, don't have the same brand on hand, want to use up something you already have, or want to experiment with a different way of preparing a meal, you can. Just be sure the food you added provides about the same number of calories as the one you took away. Use the Nutrition Facts label information to check the calorie content of packaged foods; for fresh foods, you can check the foods database at **prevention.com** or **flatbellydiet.com**. —Cynthia

Cinnamon Raisin Toast: 2 slices Food For Life® Ezekiel 4:9® Cinnamon Raisin Sprouted Bread, toasted (160), spread with ¼ cup nonfat ricotta cheese (50) and topped with 2 Tbsp **walnuts** (82); 1 medium apple (80)
■ **Total Calories = 372**

Dijon Egg Sandwich: ½ cup Organic Valley® 100% Egg Whites (50) scrambled in cooking oil spray with ¼ cup sliced red onion (23), dressed with 1 Tbsp Annie's Naturals® Organic Dijon Mustard (0), 1 slice Applegate Farms® Organic Muenster Käse Cheese (85), ½ fresh plum tomato, sliced (6), ¼ cup fresh baby spinach leaves (1), and ¼ cup sliced **avocado** (96), layered on 1 Thomas'® 100% Whole Wheat English Muffin (120)
■ **Total Calories = 381**

Farmer's Breakfast: 2 Dr. Praeger's® frozen Homestyle Potato Pancakes (150) browned in pan with 1 Tbsp **high-oleic safflower oil** (120); 2 slices cooked Applegate Farms® organic turkey bacon (60); 1 cup skim milk (80)
■ **Total Calories = 410**

Fruit & Nut Cereal: 1½ cups Kashi® 7 Whole Grain Puffs (105) with 1 cup skim milk (80), 2 Tbsp **almonds** (109), and 8 dried apricots (98)
■ **Total Calories = 392**

Mediterranean BLT: 1 Thomas'® 100% Whole Wheat English Muffin, toasted (120), spread with 2 Tbsp **black olive tapenade** (88) and 1 Laughing Cow® Mini Babybel® cheese (70); add ¼ cup sliced cucumber (5), 3 sun-dried tomatoes jarred in olive oil (30), 3 large romaine leaves (3), and 2 slices cooked Applegate Farms® organic turkey bacon (60)
■ **Total Calories = 376**

Muesli & Yogurt: 1½ cups Kashi® 7 Whole Grain Puffs (105) mixed with 6 oz Stonyfield Farm® Fat Free French Vanilla Yogurt (130) and 2 Tbsp **almonds** (109); 1 cup seedless red grapes (60)
■ **Total Calories = 404**

PB&B: 1 Thomas'® 100% Whole Wheat English Muffin, toasted (120), spread with 2 Tbsp **peanut butter** (188) and topped with ½ cup sliced banana (70)
■ **Total Calories = 378**

Peachy Pecan Oatmeal: ¾ cup dry Quaker® Old Fashioned Quick 1-Minute Oats (cooked with water to consistency of your choice) (225) mixed with 1 cup Cascadian Farm® Organic Sliced Peaches, thawed (60), and sprinkled with nutmeg and 2 Tbsp **pecans** (90)
■ **Total Calories = 375**

Peanut Butter Banana Toast: 1 slice Food For Life® Ezekiel 4:9® Sesame Sprouted Bread, toasted (80), spread with 2 Tbsp **natural creamy peanut butter** (188) and topped with ½ cup sliced banana (70); 1 cup skim milk (80)
■ **Total Calories = 418**

Peanut Butter Toast & Yogurt:

1 slice Food For Life® Ezekiel 4:9® Sprouted Sesame Bread, toasted (80), spread with 2 Tbsp **natural creamy peanut butter** (188); 1 Stonyfield Farm® Organic Lowfat Maple Vanilla Yogurt (130)

■ **Total Calories = 398**

Pecan Raisin Cereal:

1½ cups Kashi® 7 Whole Grain Puffs (105) with 1 cup skim milk (80), sprinkled with 2 Tbsp **pecans** (90) and 3 Tbsp raisins (98)

■ **Total Calories = 373**

Potato Pancakes I:

2 Dr. Praeger's® frozen Homestyle Potato Pancakes (150) browned in pan with 1 Tbsp **high-oleic safflower oil** (120); ½ cup liquid Organic Valley® 100% Egg Whites (50) scrambled with ¼ cup sliced red onion (23) and ½ fresh plum tomato, chopped (6); ½ cup 100% orange juice (55)

■ **Total Calories = 404**

Potato Pancakes II:

2 Dr. Praeger's® frozen Homestyle Potato Pancakes (150) browned in pan with 1 Tbsp **high-oleic safflower oil** (120); ½ cup liquid Organic Valley® 100% Egg Whites (50) scrambled with ¼ cup fresh chopped red bell pepper (10) and 2 Tbsp chopped scallions (4); ½ cup 100% orange juice (55)

■ **Total Calories = 389**

Raisin Almond Toast:

1 slice Food For Life® Ezekiel 4:9® Cinnamon Raisin Sprouted Bread, toasted (80), spread with 2 Tbsp **almond butter** (202); 1 cup skim milk (80); ½ cup 100% orange juice (55)

■ **Total Calories = 417**

Toasted Egg-and-Cheese Sandwich:

2 slices Fit for Life® Ezekiel 4:9® Sesame Sprouted Bread, toasted (160), spread with 1 Laughing Cow® Light Garlic & Herb Wedge (35) and filled with omelet-style egg (½ cup Organic Valley® 100% Egg Whites) (50) cooked in pan with cooking spray with ¼ cup sliced red onion (23), dressed with ½ fresh sliced plum tomato (6), 3 large romaine lettuce leaves (3), and ¼ cup sliced **avocado** (96)

■ **Total Calories = 373**

Tropical Waffle:

2 LifeStream® Organic FlaxPlus® frozen waffles, toasted (200), topped with ½ cup drained pineapple tidbits packed in juice (60) and sprinkled with cinnamon, nutmeg, and 2 Tbsp **macadamia nuts** (120)

■ **Total Calories = 380**

Vanilla Macadamia Parfait:

1½ cups Kashi® 7 Whole Grain Puffs (105) mixed with 6 oz Stonyfield Farm® Fat Free French Vanilla Yogurt (130) and 2 Tbsp **macadamia nuts** (120)

■ **Total Calories = 355**

Flat Belly Lunches

My favorite brown-bag standby: the Dijon Turkey Wrap on the next page. Yum! As with the breakfasts, MUFAs are in **boldface**, and ingredient calorie counts are in parentheses.

Boca Tacos: 4 6-inch corn tortillas, warmed (180), filled evenly with ½ cup Boca Ground Burger Crumbles, microwaved (60), and topped with ½ cup fresh baby spinach leaves (3), ¼ cup salsa (40); and ¼ cup sliced **avocado** (96) ■ **Total Calories = 379**

California Burger: 1 Boca® Original Vegan Veggie Burger (80) on 1 Food For Life® Ezekiel 4:9® Sprouted Burger Bun (150), dressed with 1 Tbsp Annie's Naturals® Organic Dijon Mustard (0), 3 large romaine lettuce leaves (3), ½ cup Roland® Roasted Red Peppers (jarred in water) (30), and ¼ cup sliced **avocado** (96) ■ **Total Calories = 359**

Chicken Lettuce Wraps I: 4 oz organic grilled chicken breast (120), glazed with 2 Tbsp China Blue® Scallion Ginger Glaze (80) and wrapped in 4 large romaine lettuce leaves (4); ½ cup fresh snow peas (20) with 2 Tbsp hummus (50) sprinkled with 2 Tbsp **pine nuts** (113), for dipping ■ **Total Calories = 387**

Chicken Lettuce Wraps II: 4 oz organic grilled chicken breast (120), chilled, brushed with 2 Tbsp China Blue® Scallion Ginger Glaze (80) and wrapped in 4 large romaine lettuce leaves (4); ½ cup fresh snow peas (20) and 2 Tbsp hummus (50) sprinkled with 2 Tbsp **pine nuts** (113), for dipping ■ **Total Calories = 387**

Cheesy Spinach Ziti: ¼ cup cooked whole wheat penne (105) tossed with 1 Tbsp **extra virgin olive oil** (119), ¼ cup nonfat ricotta cheese (50), 2 Tbsp Organic Valley® Shredded Italian Four-Cheese Blend (45), ½ cup fresh baby spinach leaves (3), 2 Tbsp sliced onions (6), and ½ cup Newman's Own® Marinara Pasta Sauce (60) ■ **Total Calories = 388**

Chilled Chicken Pasta: ¼ cup cooked and chilled whole wheat penne (105) tossed with 1 Tbsp **pesto sauce** (80), 3 oz organic precooked chicken breast, diced (90), 1 cup grape tomatoes, halved (30), ¾ cup shredded carrots (38), and 2 Tbsp Organic Valley® Shredded Italian Four-Cheese Blend (45) ■ **Total Calories = 388**

Chilled Spicy Italian Sausage Pasta: 1 Applegate Farms® Organic Sweet Italian sausage, cooked and chopped (150), tossed with ¼ cup cooked whole wheat penne, chilled (105), 1 cup grape tomatoes, halved (30), ¾ cup shredded carrots (38), and ¼ cup chopped celery (5) with 1 Tbsp **pesto sauce** (80) ■ **Total Calories = 408**

SASS FROM SASS

What about alcohol?

Whether or not you drink on the *Flat Belly Diet* is up to you. As a health care professional, my goal has always been to help people make informed decisions that work best for their own lives. So here's the information I always share regarding alcohol: Current dietary guidelines recommend that if you don't drink, you should not start. In moderation, alcohol has been shown to lower the risk of heart disease, but it also carries risks. Just one drink a day is linked to an increased risk of breast cancer, and more-than-moderate drinking is tied to liver cirrhosis, high blood pressure, cancers of the upper gastrointestinal tract, stroke, injuries, and violence.

Some people are advised not to consume alcoholic beverages at all, including pregnant and lactating women and individuals taking medications that can interact with alcohol.

That said, most adults do consume alcohol, so if you do already drink, practice moderation, meaning one drink per day for women and up to two drinks per day for men. (One drink equals 12 ounces of regular beer, 5 ounces of wine, or 1.5 ounces—one shot—of 80-proof distilled spirits.) Each of these contains about 100 calories, so to stay on track with the *Flat Belly Diet,* you'll need to balance out those calories somehow. You can either burn 100 extra calories by exercising or shave 25 calories from each of your four meals—or 50 from two. Taking 100 calories out of a single 400-calorie meal can leave you feeling too hungry, and since alcohol is an appetite stimulant, that could be a recipe for overeating.   —*Cynthia*

Crunchy Tuna Melt: 1 slice Food For Life® Ezekiel 4:9® Sesame Sprouted Bread (80) topped with 3 oz chunk light water-packed tuna (120), 2 Tbsp **sunflower seeds** (90), and 1 slice Applegate Farms provolone cheese (70), then placed under broiler or in toaster oven to melt ■ **Total Calories = 360**

Dijon Turkey Wrap: 1 Thomas'® Whole Wheat Sahara wrap (170) spread with 1 Tbsp Annie's Naturals® Organic Dijon Mustard (0), sprinkled with 2 Tbsp **pumpkin seeds** (148), and filled with 2 oz Applegate Farms® Antibiotic-free Honey Maple Turkey (50), 1/4 cup sliced red onion (23), 1/2 fresh plum tomato, sliced (6), and 3 large romaine lettuce leaves (3)

▧ **Total Calories = 400**

Dipping Trio: ²/₃ cup frozen Cascadian Farm® Organic Edamame, thawed (120), dressed with 1 Tbsp Annie's Naturals® Goddess Dressing (45); 2 Ryvita® Dark Rye Crispbread crackers (70); ½ cup organic baby carrots (25) with 2 Tbsp **tahini sauce** (178) for dipping

▧ **Total Calories = 438**

Exotic Turkey Roll-Ups: 4 oz Applegate Farms® Antibiotic-free Smoked Turkey slices (100) wrapped around 2 oz (¼ cup) Sabra™ Babaganoush (160), ½ cup sliced Roland® Roasted Red Peppers (jarred in water) (30), and 2 Tbsp **pine nuts** (113)

▧ **Total Calories = 403**

Ham & Blue Cheese Salad: 2 cups organic mixed baby greens (15) tossed with 2 Tbsp Annie's Naturals® Goddess Dressing (90) and topped with ½ fresh plum tomato, sliced (6), 3 oz Applegate Farms® uncured Black Forest ham, chopped (75), 2 Tbsp crumbled gorgonzola (50), and 2 Tbsp **pumpkin seeds** (148)

▧ **Total Calories = 384**

Italian Sausage Wraps: Sauté in 1 Tbsp **canola oil** (124): 1 Applegate Farms® Organic Sweet Italian sausage, chopped (150), ½ cup fresh chopped bell pepper (20), and ½ cup sliced red onion (46); spread evenly onto 4 large romaine leaves (4), sprinkle with 2 Tbsp crumbled gorgonzola (50), and roll up

▧ **Total Calories = 394**

Meatball Melt: 1 Thomas'® Multigrain Pita (140) filled with 3 Gardenburger® Mama Mia Veggie Meatballs (55) and 2 Tbsp Organic Valley® Shredded Italian Four-Cheese Blend (45), drizzled with 1 Tbsp **extra virgin olive oil** (119), and placed under broiler or in toaster oven to toast pita and melt cheese; ½ cup Newman's Own® Marinara Pasta Sauce (60) for dipping

▧ **Total Calories = 419**

Mediterranean Wrap: 1 Thomas'® Whole Wheat Sahara wrap (170) spread with 2 Tbsp **black olive tapenade** (88) and filled with 2 oz turkey pastrami (60), ¼ cup sliced red onion (23), ½ fresh plum tomato, sliced (6), and 3 large romaine lettuce leaves (3); side of 1 cup red grapes (60)

▧ **Total Calories = 410**

Muffuletta Wrap: 1 Thomas'® Whole Wheat Sahara wrap (170) spread with 2 Tbsp **black olive tapenade** (88) and filled with 2 oz Applegate Farms® Antibiotic-free Honey Maple Turkey (50), 1 slice Applegate Farms® provolone cheese (70), ¼ cup sliced red onion (23), ¼ cup chopped celery (5), and 3 large romaine lettuce leaves (3)

▧ **Total Calories = 409**

Niçoise Salad: 2 cups organic mixed baby greens (15) tossed with 2 Tbsp Annie's Naturals® Organic Dijon Mustard to coat (0) and topped with 1 cup skin-on red potatoes, cubed, boiled, and chilled (100), 10 sliced **large black olives** (50), ½ cup chopped green beans (15), ¼ cup chopped celery (5), ½ cup

grape tomatoes, halved (15), and 4 oz chunk light water-packed tuna (160)

■ **Total Calories = 360**

Pesto Ham & Cheese Sandwich:

1 Thomas'® 100% Whole Wheat English Muffin (120) spread with 1 Tbsp **pesto sauce** (80) and filled with 4 oz Applegate Farms uncured Black Forest ham (100), 1/2 fresh plum tomato, sliced (6), 3 large romaine leaves (3), and 1 slice Applegate Farms provolone cheese (70); 1 cup grape tomatoes (30)

■ **Total Calories = 409**

Picnic Lunch: 4 Ryvita® Dark Rye

Crispbread crackers (140) spread with 2 Tbsp Annie's Naturals® Organic Dijon Mustard (0), 13 slices Lightlife® Smart Deli Pepperoni (70), 10 **large green olives** (50), and 1/2 cup organic baby carrots (25) with 1/4 cup hummus (100) for dipping

■ **Total Calories = 385**

Shrimp Lettuce Wraps: 4 large

romaine lettuce leaves (4) filled evenly with 4 oz medium shrimp (120), glazed with 2 Tbsp China Blue® Scallion Ginger Glaze (80), broiled, chilled, and tossed with 1/4 cup chopped celery (5), 2 Tbsp minced red onion (12), 1/2 cup fresh chopped red bell pepper (20), and 2 Tbsp **cashews** (100); 1 orange (62)

■ **Total Calories = 403**

Southwest Pita Melt: 1 Thomas'®

Multigrain Pita (140) filled with 1 slice Applegate Farms® Monterey Jack with Jalapeño Peppers (70) and 1 Gardenburger® Black Bean Chipotle Veggie Burger (80)

defrosted in the microwave, then placed in toaster oven to brown pita and melt cheese and dressed with 3 large romaine lettuce leaves (3), 1/2 fresh plum tomato, sliced (6), 1/4 cup sliced **avocado** (96), and 2 Tbsp sliced onions (6)

■ **Total Calories = 401**

Southwest Veggie Burger:

1 Food For Life® Ezekiel 4:9® Sprouted Burger Bun (150) filled with 1 Gardenburger® Black Bean Chipotle Veggie Burger, microwaved (80), topped with 1/4 cup sliced **avocado** (96), 2 Tbsp sliced onions (6), 1 sliced jalapeño (4), and 1 Tbsp salsa (10); 1 medium kiwi, sliced (46)

■ **Total Calories = 392**

Spaghetti & Meatballs: 1/4 cup

cooked whole wheat spaghetti (105) tossed with 1 Tbsp **extra virgin olive oil** (119) and topped with 1/2 cup Newman's Own® Marinara Pasta Sauce (60) and 6 Gardenburger® Mama Mia Veggie Meatballs, mirowaved (110)

■ **Total Calories = 394**

Spinach Black Bean Wrap:

1 Thomas'® Whole Wheat Sahara Wrap (170) filled with 1 Gardenburger® Black Bean Chipotle Veggie Burger, microwaved and chopped (80), and topped with 1/2 cup fresh baby spinach leaves (3), 2 Tbsp chopped scallions (4), and 1/4 cup sliced **avocado** (96)

■ **Total Calories = 353**

Tuna Pita: Half of a Thomas'® Multigrain Pita (70) filled with 3 ounces chunk light tuna in water (120), 2 diced sun-dried tomatoes jarred in extra virgin olive oil (20), 2 Tbsp chopped **walnuts** (82), and 2 Tbsp crumbled feta cheese (60)

▧ **Total Calories = 352**

Tuna Salad: 2 cups organic mixed baby greens (15) tossed with 2 Tbsp Newman's Own® Light Balsamic Vinaigrette (45) and topped with 3 oz chunk light water-packed tuna (120), 2 Tbsp **walnuts** (82), and 1 oz crumbled feta cheese (80); 1 plum (30)

▧ **Total Calories = 372**

Turkey Cranberry Muffin:

1 Thomas'® 100% Whole Wheat English Muffin (120) spread with 1 Laughing Cow® Light Garlic & Herb Wedge (35) and filled with 3 oz Applegate Farms® Antibiotic-free Honey Maple Turkey (75), 1 Tbsp dried cranberries (45), and 2 Tbsp **walnuts** (82)

▧ **Total Calories = 357**

Waldorf Pita: 1 Thomas'® Multigrain Pita (140) spread with 2 wedges Laughing Cow® Light Swiss Original (70) and filled with ¼ cup chopped celery (5), 1 medium apple, sliced (80), 2 Tbsp **walnuts** (82), and 3 large romaine lettuce leaves (3)

▧ **Total Calories = 380**

SASS FROM SASS

"You Are Better Off with Breakfast!"

When I was a dietitian in private practice, at least once a week someone would tell me that they "do better" when they skip breakfast. Unfortunately, this isn't true for anybody, and research proves it. In fact, a whopping 78 percent of successful dieters registered with the National Weight Control registry, a database of individuals who've lost 30 pounds or more and have kept it off for at least a year, eat breakfast. What about the theory that skipping this meal is a natural way to eliminate calories? Studies show that breakfast skippers make up for those calories by unknowingly eating more later in the day. Some of my clients swore that eating breakfast made them hungrier. Well, in fact, eating breakfast does stimulate your appetite because it kicks your metabolism into high gear. A faster metabolism means a flatter belly and more calories burned all day long, so overall, you are better off with breakfast. —*Cynthia*

Flat Belly Dinners

Don't hesitate to whip up additional portions of these dinners for your family. Our testers raved and were so thankful that these options pleased husbands, kids, and teens alike! As with breakfasts and lunches, MUFAs are in **boldface**, and ingredient calorie counts are in parentheses.

California Turkey Salad: 2 cups organic mixed baby greens (15) tossed with 2 Tbsp Newman's Own® Light Balsamic Vinaigrette (45) and topped with 3 oz browned all-breast-meat ground turkey (130), 2 Tbsp crumbled gorgonzola (50), and 2 Tbsp **walnuts** (82); 1 small pear (86)
■ Total Calories = 408

Cheesy Veggie Pasta: ¼ cup fresh chopped red bell peppers (10), ½ cup broccoli florets (20), and 2 Tbsp sliced onions (6) sautéed in 1 Tbsp **extra virgin olive oil** (119) and tossed with ¼ cup nonfat ricotta cheese (50), 2 Tbsp Organic Valley® Shredded Italian Four-Cheese Blend (45), and ¼ cup cooked whole wheat penne (105)
■ Total Calories = 355

Chicago-Style Hot Dog: 1 Lightlife® Jumbo Smart Dog (45), browned in skillet in 1 Tbsp **peanut oil** (119), on 1 Food For Life® Ezekiel 4:9® Sprouted Hot Dog Bun (170) dressed with 1 Tbsp mustard (0), 2 Tbsp diced onions (6), 2 Tbsp sweet relish (30), ½ fresh tomato, diced (6), and a dash of celery seed
■ Total Calories = 376

Chicken Caesar: 2 cups organic mixed baby greens (15) tossed with 1 Tbsp **olive oil** (124) and 1 Tbsp Newman's Own Lighten Up Caesar dressing (35) and topped with 3 oz organic precooked chicken breast (90), chilled (optional: sear on grill); 1 oz Asiago cheese (103); and 1 Ryvita Dark Rye Crispbread cracker (35).
■ Total Calories = 402

Chicken Caprese: 2 oz organic grilled chicken breast (60) served with ½ cup steamed wild rice (150) and tomato mozzarella salad made with 1 plum tomato, sliced (12), 1 oz sliced Polly-O® Part-Skim Mozzarella (70), and 2 fresh basil leaves (0) drizzled with 1 Tbsp **olive oil** (124) and 1 Tbsp balsamic vinegar (5), and dusted with cracked black pepper
■ Total Calories = 421

Edamame Salad: 2 cups organic mixed baby greens (15) tossed with 2 Tbsp Annie's Naturals® Goddess Dressing (90) and topped with ⅔ cup Cascadian Farm® Organic Edamame, thawed (120), ½ cup canned mandarin oranges, drained (80), and 2 Tbsp **almonds** (109)
■ Total Calories = 414

Edamame Wild Rice Salad: ¼ cup

cooked wild rice (75), chilled, tossed with ½ cup Cascadian Farm® Organic Edamame, thawed (90), 1 cup Cascadian Farm® Organic Chinese Stir-Fry vegetables, thawed (25), 2 Tbsp Annie's Naturals® Goddess Dressing (90), and 2 Tbsp **cashews** (100)

▨ **Total Calories = 380**

Grilled Chicken Salad: 2 cups

organic mixed baby greens (15) tossed with 2 Tbsp balsamic vinegar (10) and 1 Tbsp **extra virgin olive oil** (119) and topped with 3 oz organic grilled chicken breast (90), ½ cup broccoli florets (20), ¾ cup shredded carrots (38), ¼ cup sliced red onion (23), ¾ cup Cascadian Farm® Organic Sweet Corn, thawed (70), and freshly ground black pepper

▨ **Total Calories = 385**

Grilled Pork Salad: 3 oz pork

tenderloin, grilled (115), served on a bed of 2 cups organic mixed baby greens (15) tossed with ½ cup drained pineapple tidbits (60), ¼ cup fresh chopped red bell peppers (10), ¼ cup crumbled feta (80), 2 Tbsp balsamic vinegar (10), and 1 Tbsp **extra virgin olive oil** (119)

▨ **Total Calories = 409**

Mexicali Salad: 2 cups organic

mixed baby greens (15) topped with ½ cup Amy's® Organic Refried Beans with Green Chiles (130), ¾ cup Cascadian Farm® Organic Sweet Corn, thawed (70), ¼ cup sliced red onion (23), ¼ cup salsa (40), and ¼ cup sliced **avocado** (96)

▨ **Total Calories = 374**

Pepperoni Pizza: 1 flat Thomas'®

Multigrain Pita (140) brushed on one side with 1 Tbsp **extra virgin olive oil** (119) and topped with ¼ cup Newman's Own® Marinara Pasta Sauce (30), 13 slices Lightlife® Smart Deli Pepperoni (40), and 2 Tbsp Organic Valley® Shredded Italian Four-Cheese Blend (45); warm under broiler or in toaster oven to heat through

▨ **Total Calories = 374**

Pineapple-Ham Pizza: 1 flat

Thomas'® Multigrain Pita (140) brushed on one side with 1 Tbsp **extra virgin olive oil** (119) and topped with ¼ cup Newman's Own® Marinara Pasta Sauce (30), ¼ cup drained pineapple tidbits (30), ¼ cup fresh chopped red bell peppers (10), 2 oz Applegate Farms® uncured Black Forest ham, chopped (50), and 2 Tbsp crumbled gorgonzola (50); warm under broiler or in toaster oven to heat through

▨ **Total Calories = 429**

Pork with Szechuan Vegetables:

2 cups Cascadian Farm® Organic Chinese Stir-Fry vegetables (50) sautéed in 1 Tbsp **canola oil** (124) flavored with ground szechuan peppercorns and served with 3 oz pork tenderloin, sliced (115), and ½ cup cooked Uncle Ben's® Ready Brown Rice (110)

▨ **Total Calories = 399**

Ricotta Calzone: 1/4 cup nonfat ricotta cheese (50) mixed with 2 sundried tomatoes jarred in olive oil, diced (20), 1 Tbsp **extra virgin olive oil** (119), 1 tsp minced garlic (10), and 4 fresh basil leaves, sliced (0), and stuffed into 1 Thomas'® Multigrain Pita (140); warm under broiler until pita is golden and cheeses are bubbly; serve with 1/2 cup Newman's Own® Marinara Pasta Sauce (60) for dipping
▨ **Total Calories = 399**

Salmon Pistachio Lettuce Wraps: 4 large romaine lettuce leaves (4) filled evenly with 1/4 cup dill hummus (100), 1/2 cup canned Alaskan salmon (180), 1/2 fresh plum tomato, diced (6), 1/4 cup diced cucumber (5), and 2 Tbsp **pistachios** (88)
▨ **Total Calories = 383**

Salmon Sandwich: 2 slices Food For Life® Ezekiel 4:9® Sesame Sprouted Bread (160) spread with 2 Tbsp **black olive tapenade** (88), 1/2 cup canned Alaskan salmon (180), 1/2 fresh plum tomato, diced (6), and 2 large romaine lettuce leaves (2)
▨ **Total Calories = 436**

SASS FROM SASS

"Take a Lunch Break!"

A recent survey found that a whopping 74 percent of American office workers eat lunch at their desks. Eating while working can cause you to eat too fast, lose track of how much you've eaten, and distract you from the taste and enjoyment of your meal. Follow these lunchtime rules to help make your midday meal a priority.

Set your cell phone or computer alarm to remind you to stop and eat. When it goes off, don't hit the snooze or dismiss it. You can pick up where you left off after your meal feeling reenergized.

Commit to eating lunch with a co-worker. When you know a friend is waiting for you, you won't talk yourself into staying at your desk.

Use real dishes and silverware. In Europe (where the average lunchtime is 50 percent longer but waistlines are smaller), people in France, Greece, Italy, Portugal, Spain, and other countries rely on this tradition to make each meal feel special. Store a set in your office kitchen—washing them will tack just a few seconds onto your meal.

If you really have to eat at your desk, try not to work while you eat. Take a few deep breaths, and savor every bite—even if it's only for 10 minutes.
—*Cynthia*

Salmon Steak Almondine: 4 oz grilled wild Alaskan salmon (215) served with 1½ cups frozen Cascadian Farm® Organic Cut Green Beans, steamed or microwaved (60), and dressed with freshly ground white pepper and 2 Tbsp **sliced almonds** (109)
▓ **Total Calories = 384**

Savory Turkey Pasta: ½ cup broccoli florets (20) and 1 cup plum tomato, sliced (30), sautéed in 1 Tbsp **extra virgin olive oil** (119) and tossed with 4 fresh basil leaves, sliced (0), 3 oz browned all-breast-meat ground turkey (130), and ¼ cup cooked whole wheat penne (105)
▓ **Total Calories = 404**

Sesame Ginger Shrimp Wrap:
1 Thomas'® Whole Wheat Sahara wrap (170) filled with 3 oz broiled medium shrimp (90), ¼ cup fresh snow peas (10), ¼ cup chopped celery (5), and 2 Tbsp **cashews** (100) and drizzled with 1 Tbsp Newman's Own® Lighten Up Low Fat Sesame Ginger Dressing (18)
▓ **Total Calories = 393**

Shrimp and Snow Pea Sesame Pasta: 2 oz medium broiled shrimp (60), chilled, and ¼ cup cooked, chilled whole wheat spirals (105) tossed with 1 Tbsp **sesame oil** (120), ¼ cup fresh snow peas (10), 2 Tbsp chopped scallions (4), and ¼ cup chopped celery (5) and sprinkled with 1 Tbsp whole black sesame seeds (50)
▓ **Total Calories = 354**

Slaw Dog: 1 Lightlife® Jumbo Smart Dog (45) browned in skillet in 1 Tbsp **peanut oil** (119), on 1 Food For Life® Ezekiel 4:9® Sprouted Hot Dog Bun (170) dressed with 1 Tbsp mustard (0) and half of a 12-ounce bag of Mann's® Broccoli Coleslaw mix (50) tossed with 2 Tbsp Newman's Own® Light Balsamic Vinaigrette (45)
▓ **Total Calories = 429**

Spicy Shrimp: 3 oz medium shrimp (90), brushed with 1 Tbsp China Blue® Spicy Chili Bean Glaze (40) and grilled, served with ½ cup steamed wild rice (150) and 1 cup fresh asparagus (30) sautéed in 1 Tbsp **canola oil** (124), 1 tsp minced garlic jarred in water (10), 1 Tbsp fresh chopped parsley (0), and freshly ground black pepper
▓ **Total Calories = 444**

Spinach Burrito: 1 Thomas'® Whole Wheat Sahara wrap (170) filled with ½ cup fresh spinach (3), 1 tsp minced garlic (10), and ¼ cup sliced red onion (12) sautéed in 1 Tbsp **olive oil** (119) and topped with 1 oz Asiago Fresco cheese (103)
▓ **Total Calories = 417**

Szechuan Chicken: 2 cups frozen Cascadian Farm® Organic Chinese Stir-Fry vegetables (50) sautéed in 1 Tbsp **canola oil** (124) flavored with ground szechuan peppercorns, served with 3 oz organic grilled chicken breast (90) and ½ cup cooked Uncle Ben's® Ready Brown Rice (110)
▓ **Total Calories = 374**

Turkey Quesadilla: Spread 1 Laughing Cow® Light Garlic & Herb Wedge (35) on 1 Thomas'® Whole Wheat Sahara wrap (170). On half of wrap, place 2 oz Applegate Farms® Antibiotic-free Honey Maple Turkey (50), ¼ cup baby spinach leaves (1), 2 Tbsp crumbled feta (40), and 10 sliced **large black olives** (50). Fold over and heat in toaster oven or a nonstick pan over medium heat.
■ **Total Calories = 346**

Turkey Sauté: ½ cup fresh chopped red bell pepper (20) and ¼ cup sliced red onion (23) sautéed in 1 Tbsp **olive oil** (119), tossed with 2 Tbsp chopped scallions (4), 4 fresh basil leaves, sliced (0), and 3 oz browned all-breast-meat ground turkey (130), served with 3 oz (⅕ of bag) Alexia® Oven Fries with Olive Oil, Rosemary & Garlic, cooked under broiler or in toaster oven (120)
■ **Total Calories = 416**

Turkey Tacos: Sauté ¼ cup chopped red bell pepper (10) and 2 Tbsp sliced red onion (12) in 1 Tbsp **olive oil** (119). Brown 3 oz all-breast-meat ground turkey (130). Fill 3 6-inch corn tortillas (135) evenly with turkey, then add pepper mixture and sprinkle with 2 Tbsp chopped scallions (4) and ¼ cup shredded carrots (14).
■ **Total Calories = 424**

Wild Salmon Cashew Salad:
2 cups organic mixed baby greens (15) tossed with 2 Tbsp Newman's Own® Lighten Up Low Fat Sesame Ginger Dressing (35) and topped with 4 oz grilled wild Alaskan salmon (215) and 2 Tbsp **cashews** (100)
■ **Total Calories = 365**

MEAL REPLACEMENT BARS

CHOOSE 1 OF THE FOLLOWING MEAL REPLACEMENT BARS	CALORIES	ADD YOUR MUFA
Clif® Black Cherry Almond Bar	250	
Clif® Crunchy Peanut Butter Bar	250	
Odwalla® Chocolate Chip Peanut bar	250	
Clif® Chocolate Brownie bar	240	Add 1 piece of fruit and a 100- to 150-calorie MUFA from the list on page 101, such as 2 Tbsp of (choose 1): ■ almonds (109) ■ Brazil nuts (110) ■ peanuts (110) ■ macadamia nuts (120) OR Add a 150- to 200-calorie MUFA from the list on page 101, such as 2 Tbsp of (choose 1): ■ natural peanut butter (188) ■ almond butter (200)
Odwalla® Banana Nut bar	240	
Nature's Path® Optimum® Pomegran Cherry energy bar	230	
Larabar® Chocolate Coconut	220	
Larabar® Banana Bread	220	
Larabar® Ginger Snap	220	
Larabar® Cinnamon Roll	210	
Nature's Path® Optimum® Blueberry Flax & Soy energy bar	200	
Larabar® Pecan Pie	200	
Nature's Path® Optimum® Cranberry Zen energy bar	200	
Larabar® Cherry Pie	190	
Larabar® Apple Pie	180	
Luna® Chai Tea bar	180	
Luna® Chocolate Pecan Pie bar	180	
Luna® Lemon Zest bar	180	
Luna® Nutz Over Chocolate™ bar	180	
Luna® Peanut Butter Cookie bar	180	
Luna® S'mores bar	180	

FROZEN MEALS

CHOOSE 1 OF THE FOLLOWING MEALS	CALORIES	ADD YOUR MUFA
Amy's® Chili & Cornbread Dinner	340	Add a 50- to 100-calorie MUFA from the list on page 101, such as: ■ 10 large green or black olives (or 5 of each) (50)
Kashi® Black Bean Mango	340	
Amy's® Black Bean Enchilada Dinner	330	
Kashi® Lemon Rosemary Chicken	330	
Amy's® Indian Mattar Paneer	320	
Kashi® Sweet & Sour Chicken	320	
Seeds of Change® Moroccan LentiTagine	320	
Amy's® Indian Vegetable Korma	300	
Seeds of Change® Hanalei Vegetarian Chicken Teriyaki	300	
Amy's® Organic Brown Rice, Black-Eyed Peas & Veggies Bowl	290	
Amy's® Organic Teriyaki Bowl	280	Add a 100- to 150-calorie MUFA from the list on page 101, such as 2 Tbsp of (choose 1): ■ almonds (109) ■ peanuts (110) ■ pumpkin seeds (148)
Amy's® Veggie Loaf Dinner	280	
Kashi® Chicken Pasta Pomodoro	280	
Seeds of Change® Lasagna Calabrese with Eggplant and Portobello Mushrooms	270	
Amy's® Indian Mattar Tofu	260	
Kashi® Lime Cilantro Shrimp	250	
Gardenburger® Black Bean Chipotle Wrap	240	
Gardenburger® Margherita Pizza Wrap	240	
Kashi® Southwest Style Chicken	240	
Cedarlane™ Low Fat Veggie Pizza Wrap	220	Add a 150- to 200-calorie MUFA from the list on page 101, such as: ■ ¼ cup chocolate chips (207)
Yves® Meatless Penne	210	
Amy's Light in Sodium Shepherd's Pie	160	
Boca® Meatless Chili	150	

FAST FOOD

MENU ITEM(S)	CALORIES	ADD YOUR MUFA
McDonald's® Premium Asian Salad with Grilled Chicken and Newman's Own® Low-Fat Sesame Ginger Dressing	390	Add a 50- to 100-calorie MUFA from the list on page 101, such as:
Baja Fresh® Baja Ensalada with Charbroiled Chicken with Salsa	325	
Jack in the Box® Asian Grilled Chicken Salad with Roasted Slivered Almonds and Low-Fat Balsamic Dressing	310	▪ 10 large green or black olives (or 5 of each) (50)
Pizza Hut® Fit n' Delicious™ Pizza (two slices) with Green pepper, Red Onion & Diced Tomato (12″)	280	▪ 2 Tbsp walnuts (82)
Fazoli's® Chicken and Fruit Salad with Fat-Free Honey Mustard	280	▪ 2 Tbsp pistachios (89)
Arby's® Junior Roast Beef Sandwich	273	▪ 2 Tbsp sunflower seeds (90)
Chick-fil-A® Chargrilled Chicken Sandwich	270	
Jamba Juice® Berry Fulfilling® smoothie (24 oz)	260	Add a 100- to 150-calorie MUFA from the list on page 101, such as:
Boston Market® roasted turkey breast (180) with poultry gravy (15) and steamed vegetables (60)	255	
Taco Bell® Chicken Enchirito® (Fresco Style)	240	▪ 2 Tbsp pumpkin seeds (148)
Wendy's® Small Chili	220	
Panera® Low-Fat Vegetarian Garden Vegetable Soup (8 oz) with a Whole Grain Loaf	220	
Au Bon Pain® Jamaican Black Bean Soup (medium)	180	Add a 150- to 200-calorie MUFA from the list on page 101, such as 2 Tbsp of (choose 1):
Taco Bell® Ranchero Chicken Soft Taco (Fresco Style)	170	
Subway® Oven Roasted Chicken Salad with Fat Free Italian Dressing and Roasted Chicken Noodle Soup	175 / 80	▪ natural peanut butter (188)
Panda Express® String Bean Chicken Breast with Mixed Vegetables	160 / 90	▪ almond butter (200)
Domino's® Grilled Chicken Caesar with Light Italian Dressing	125	

Snack Pack Options

There are 28 Snack Pack choices to choose from. You will see 10 sweet options, 10 savory options, 4 grab-and-go choices, and 4 smoothies. MUFAs are in **boldface**.

YOU CAN HAVE ONE SNACK PACK to "spend" per day.

PLAN YOUR SNACK PACK IN ADVANCE. I recommend carving out about 10 minutes each night to think through your schedule for the following day. You should decide where in the day you'll "place" your Snack Pack based on what you have planned. You may need to pack it the night before and bring it with you so you'll have it ready when you need it.

YOU CAN EAT THE SNACK PACK either between breakfast and lunch, between lunch and dinner, or between dinner and bedtime—whichever is best for your schedule. I just ask that you use it to ensure that you do not go more than 4 to 5 hours without eating. The goal is to use the Snack Pack to keep your energy and blood sugar steady, keep your metabolism revved up, and prevent your hunger from getting out of control (which often results in rebound overeating).

Sweet

Blueberry-Almond Oatmeal:

1 packet plain instant oatmeal, cooked, topped with 1½ cups blueberries and 2 Tbsp **almonds**, 1 cup skim milk
■ **Total Calories = 384**

Chocolate-Raspberry Oatmeal:

1 packet plain instant oatmeal, cooked, topped with 1 cup raspberries and ¼ cup **semisweet chocolate chips**
■ **Total Calories = 367**

Tropical-Nut Oatmeal: 1 packet

pain instant oatmeal, cooked, topped with 1 cup canned pineapple and 2 Tbsp **macadamia nuts**, 1 cup skim milk
■ **Total Calories = 420**

PB&A Oatmeal: 2 Tbsp **peanut butter**

swirled into 1 packet plain instant oatmeal, cooked, and topped with 1 medium sliced apple
■ **Total Calories = 368**

Apple Snack: 1 medium apple cut into

wedges with 2 Tbsp **peanut butter** as a dip, and 4 cups light microwaved popcorn
■ **Total Calories = 368**

Pineapple "Sundae": 1 cup canned

pineapple mixed into 1 cup nonfat cottage cheese, sprinkled with 2 Tbsp **walnuts**
■ **Total Calories = 344**

Strawberry-Chocolate "Sundae": 1 cup sliced strawberries

and ¼ cup **semisweet chocolate chips** mixed into ½ cup cottage cheese
■ **Total Calories = 347**

PB&A Muffin: 1 100% whole wheat English muffin spread with 2 Tbsp **peanut butter**, topped with 1 medium sliced apple
- **Total Calories = 388**

Apples & Crackers: 3 Ry Krisp® crackers spread with 2 Tbsp **almond butter**, topped or eaten with 1 medium sliced apple
- **Total Calories = 387**

Berry-Nut Whip: 2 cups sliced strawberries and 2 Tbsp **peanuts** mixed into 6 oz (80-calorie) vanilla yogurt
- **Total Calories = 363**

Savory

Hummus Dip: ½ cup hummus sprinkled with 2 Tbsp **pine nuts** served with 1 cup red pepper slices
- **Total Calories = 403**

Deli Snack: 3 Ry Krisp® crackers spread with 2 Tbsp **black olive tapenade**, 1 cup grape tomatoes, and 4 oz organic deli turkey slices
- **Total Calories = 323**

Cheesy Black Bean Dip: ½ cup canned black beans, rinsed, drained, and mashed, topped with ¼ cup chopped **avocado**, and sprinkled with 1 chopped low-fat string cheese. Serve with 1 cup baby carrots
- **Total Calories = 316**

Black Bean Dip 'n' Tomatoes: ½ cup canned black beans, rinsed, drained, and mashed, and mixed with 1 cup halved grape tomatoes, topped with ¼ cup chopped **avocado**, and sprinkled with 1 chopped string cheese and served with 3 Ry Krisp® crackers
- **Total Calories = 401**

Open-Faced Turkey Sandwich: 1 100% whole wheat English muffin spread with 2 Tbsp **green olive tapenade**, topped with 4 oz organic deli turkey and 1 cup canned (water-packed) artichoke hearts, drained
- **Total Calories = 344**

Open-Faced Tomato Sandwich: 1 100% whole wheat English muffin spread with 1 cup cottage cheese and 1 cup halved grape tomatoes and sprinkled with 2 Tbsp **pine nuts**
- **Total Calories = 405**

Cheese & Crackers: ½ cup cottage cheese mixed with 1 cup chopped red pepper, 1 tsp salt-free Italian seasoning, and 10 sliced large **black olives** served with 6 Ry Krisp® crackers
- **Total Calories = 380**

Deli Wrap: 4 oz organic deli turkey slices filled with ¼ cup **hummus**, sprinkled with 2 Tbsp pine nuts, and rolled up
- **Total Calories = 391**

Turkey Roll: 4 oz organic deli turkey slices filled with ¼ cup chopped **avocado**, 1 chopped low-fat string cheese, and 1 cup red pepper strips and rolled up
- **Total Calories = 316**

Pesto Chicken Wrap: 4 oz deli chicken slices filled with mixture of ½ cup cottage cheese and 1 Tbsp **pesto**, topped with 1 cup halved grape tomatoes and 1 cup canned (water-packed) artichoke hearts, drained and rolled up
- **Total Calories = 360**

Grab & Go

Option 1: 1 low-fat string cheese, 1 cup pineapple fruit cup (in juice), 1 cup baby carrots, and 2 Tbsp **peanuts**
- **Total Calories = 340**

Option 2: 1 low-fat string cheese, 4 cups popped light microwave popcorn, ¼ cup grated Parmesan, and 2 Tbsp **sunflower seeds**
- **Total Calories = 378**

Option 3: 6 oz (80-calorie) yogurt, 1 medium apple, 2 Tbsp **Brazil nuts**, and 1 cup skim milk
- **Total Calories = 350**

Option 4: 6 oz (80-calorie) yogurt, 1 medium orange, and 2 Tbsp **almonds**
- **Total Calories = 259**

Smoothies

Blueberry: Blend 1 cup skim or soy milk, 6 oz (80-calorie) vanilla yogurt, and 1 cup fresh blueberries plus a handful of ice OR 1 cup frozen blueberries for 1 minute. Transfer to a glass, and stir in 1 Tbsp organic cold-pressed **flaxseed oil**
- **Total Calories = 360**

Chocolate-Raspberry: Blend ½ cup skim or soy milk, 6 oz (80-calorie) vanilla yogurt, ¼ cup **semisweet chocolate chips**, and 1 cup fresh raspberries plus a handful of ice OR 1 cup frozen raspberries for 1 minute. Transfer to a glass, and eat with a spoon
- **Total Calories = 387**

Lemon: Blend 1 cup skim or soy milk, 6 oz (80-calorie) lemon yogurt, 1 medium orange, sliced into sections, and a handful of ice for 1 minute. Transfer to a glass, and stir in 1 Tbsp organic cold-pressed **flaxseed oil**
- **Total Calories = 370**

Apple Pie: Blend ½ cup skim or soy milk, 6 oz (80-calorie) vanilla yogurt, 1 tsp apple pie spice, 1 medium apple, peeled, cored, and chopped, 2 Tbsp **cashew butter**, and a handful of ice for 1 minute. Transfer to a glass, and eat with a spoon
- **Total Calories = 388**

Create Your Own Snack Pack

KEEP THE TOTAL CALORIE COUNT UNDER 400, INCLUDE A SELECTION FROM THE MUFA LIST ON PAGE 101, AND PAIR WITH THE FOLLOWING FOODS.

SOME MUFA CHOICES:

- 10 olives
- 1 cup soybeans
- ¼ cup avocado
- ¼ cup semisweet chocolate chips
- 2 Tbsp nuts or seeds
- 2 Tbsp olive tapenade
- 1 Tbsp oil

Please consult the full chart on page 101

GRAINS

Corn tortillas—2—90 calories

Dr. Praeger's® frozen Homestyle Potato Pancakes—1—75 calories

Food For Life® Ezekiel Cinnamon Raisin Sprouted Grain Bread—1 slice—80 calories

Food For Life Ezekiel Sesame Sprouted Grain Bread—1 slice—80 calories

Kashi® 7 Whole Grain Puffs—1 cup—70 calories

Lifestream® Organic Flax Plus frozen waffle—1—100 calories

Oatmeal—1 (1 oz) packet instant plain—100 calories

Popcorn—4 cups light microwave (a brand that provides 20-25 calories per cup popped, such as Wild Oats® organic plain popcorn, Smart Balance® Light, or Newman's Own® 94% fat free)—100 calories

Ry Krisp® crackers—3—75 calories

Thomas'® multigrain pita—½—70 calories

Thomas'® 100% whole wheat English muffin—1 whole—120 calories

Uncle Ben's® Ready Brown Rice—½ cup—110 calories

DAIRY

Applegate Farms® Monterey Jack with Jalapeño Peppers—1 slice—70 calories

Applegate Farms® provolone cheese—1 slice—70 calories

Cottage cheese, nonfat—½ cup—80 calories

Feta cheese—1 oz—80 calories

Milk, skim or unsweetened—1 cup—80 calories

Organic Valley® Shredded Italian Four-Cheese Blend—1/4 cup—90 calories

String cheese, low-fat (1 oz)—80 calories

Yogurt, nonfat (6 oz)—80 calories

FRUITS

Apple, any variety, medium (size of a tennis ball)—80 calories

Berries (blueberries, raspberries, or strawberries)—1 cup—60 calories

Frozen Cascadian Farm® Organic Pitted Dark Sweet Cherries—1 cup—100 calories

Kiwi—1 cup sliced—110 calories

Mango—1 cup sliced—110 calories

Mott's® Natural Style Unsweetened Apple Sauce—1 cup—100 calories

Orange, medium—70 calories

Papaya—1 cup cubed—55 calories

Peach—1 medium—50 calories

Pear—1 medium—100 calories

Pineapple, canned in pineapple juice—4 oz or 1/2 cup—60 calories

Plums—2 medium—60 calories

Red or green grapes—1 cup—60 calories

Sliced banana—1/2 cup—70 calories

Unsweetened raisins—1/4 cup—130 calories

Watermelon—2 cups diced—90 calories

VEGETABLES

Artichoke hearts, canned in water—1 cup—70 calories

Baby carrots—1 cup—50 calories

Broccoli florets, raw—2 cups—40 calories

Cauliflower florets, raw—2 cups—50 calories

Grape tomatoes—1 cup—30 calories

Mann's® Broccoli Coleslaw mix—12 ounce bag—50 calories

Newman's Own® Marinara Pasta Sauce—1/2 cup—60 calories

Organic mixed baby greens—2 cups—15 calories

Radishes—1 cup sliced—20 calories

Red (bell) pepper, sliced—1 cup—40 calories

Salsa—1/4 cup—40 calories

PROTEINS

Applegate Farms® uncured Black Forest ham—4 oz—100 calories

Black beans, canned, drained—1/2 cup—90 calories

Boca® Original Vegan veggie burger—1—80 calories

Chunk light tuna in water—3 oz—120 calories

Deli chicken slices—4 oz—100 calories

Deli turkey slices—4 oz—100 calories

Gardenburger® Black Bean Chipotle Veggie Burger—1—80 calories

Gardenburger® Mama Mia veggie meatballs—6—110 calories

Hummus—1/4 cup—100 calories

Organic precooked chicken breast—3 oz—90 calories

READ A FLAT BELLY
SUCCESS
STORY

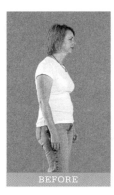

BEFORE

AFTER

Julie Plavsic

AGE: 42

POUNDS LOST:

6

IN 32 DAYS

ALL-OVER
INCHES LOST:

6.5

I HAD A BABY A COUPLE OF YEARS AGO AND SINCE THEN—until now, anyway—I've been struggling with 10 stubborn pounds. I was on the lower end of what I needed to lose, but I just couldn't get the scale to budge. I was eating healthy . . . exercising . . . nothing seemed to be working. Of course, I have to confess, I didn't have the most perfect eating habits at the time."

Julie admits to many of the behaviors that lead to a dieter's downfall. She was grazing on "stuff" all day long, she says. And she wasn't always honest with herself about what and how much she was eating. "Like pasta. I was having what I thought was a small serving of pasta, but according to the *Flat Belly Diet,* I was actually having a double or a triple portion. Who really measures? It looked like a small portion, so I told myself it was fine."

At first, looking at 1,600 calories a day, she didn't think she could do it. But it wasn't hard, she claims, because the food is so filling. The MUFAs amazed her. She tried dozens of things on the menu the first couple of weeks, but in the end, she needed to simplify. With a job as an immigration lawyer and a small baby, Julie needed meals that she could create quickly. "So I ended up having the same thing every morning—

peanut butter on toast—which I love. And after that, I was full until lunch. No more snacking all morning."

What was hard for her, she claims, was changing her thinking in so many ways. "I knew that the diet required us to eat things like olives and olive oil. And even though I knew that the calories were not that bad, it was hard at first for me to believe that you can fight fat by eating fat. Or that fat has to do with other things as well. I had to get over all those years of denying myself those high-fat foods. It was a leap of faith."

It was a leap she's glad she took. "I learned so much from this diet," she says. "First of all, I learned that belly fat can be more dangerous than the other kinds of fat, and so with this diet, I'm making my body healthier in addition to making it thinner. I also learned that what the scale says is so much less important than how you feel. I wanted to get to 130, but I'm happy with how I look and how my clothes fit at 133."

Julie doesn't consider what she's doing a "diet," per se. For her, it's more a new way of looking at food, of making choices and using calories wisely, a way of portioning out what you need to put in each meal throughout the day. "I'm thinking about all the overweight friends I have," she says. "I'm so excited by this diet, I can't *wait* to get them to try it!"

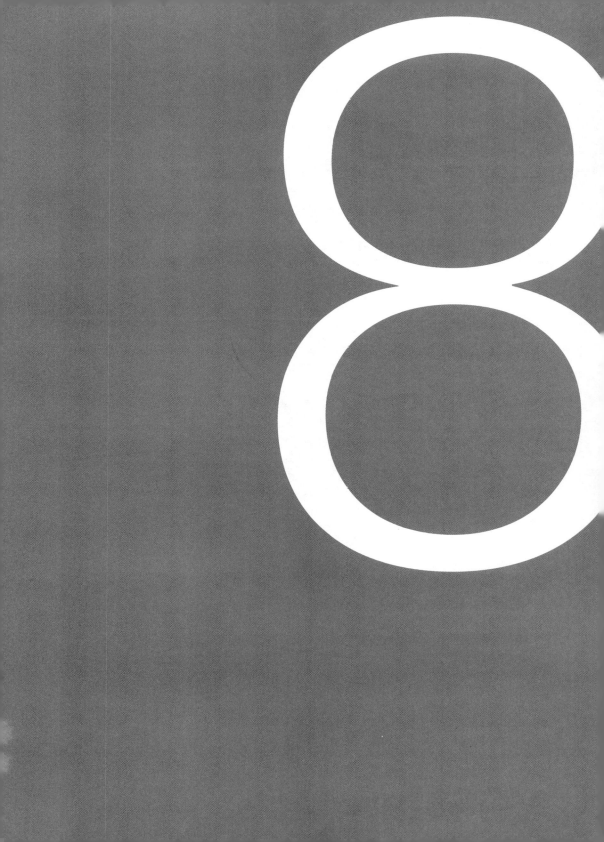

THE FOUR-WEEK PLAN: RECIPES

I HAVE A CONFESSION TO MAKE. I'm not a big cook. I have my
specialties (well, specialty: an hors d'oeuvre of mini pumpernickel
slices spread with a melted Cheddar, olive, and curry mixture) that
I rely on whenever I have company, but for the most part, my husband's the chef in the house. He's also, bless his heart, the one who
does most of the grocery shopping. I'm good at saying what I like
(helpfully encouraging him to make things that are fresh, healthy,
vegetable-filled, and filling) and what would be better served when
I'm away on a business trip.

Now why, you're probably wondering, would Liz start off the recipe
chapter with a confession like that? Because I vowed that any recipe
chapter in a book of mine needed to be filled with dishes I could
envision myself making. If I see a recipe that has a dozen or more

ingredients and takes a day to prepare, my eyes glaze over and I start thinking about ordering a pizza.

To that end, the recipes you'll find here are sufficiently gourmet to make your mouth water and get your creative chef juices flowing. But they're also extremely simple. Take the Pumpkin Spiced Oatmeal on page 150. *It takes 2 minutes! (My kinda recipe, that!)* Or the Sweet-and-Sour Shrimp on page 205—a mere 15 minutes start to finish. And believe me, the flavors will astound you.

But what really makes these recipes extraordinary is not how easy or fast they are to prepare but how well they fit into the *Flat Belly Diet*. Each serving contains a MUFA, for starters. As you know, MUFAs are the only foods that can specifically help reduce belly fat. You can spot them in the ingredient lists; they're in **boldface**. In addition, beside most recipes is a very important component titled "Make It a Flat Belly Diet Meal." This box tells you what to add to one serving of that recipe to turn it into a meal that you can slot right into your menu plan. Let's say you decide to start your day with a serving of the delicious Apple Pancakes on page 148. Your MUFA is included. But remember that every meal on the *Flat Belly Diet* should equal roughly 400 calories. When you sit down to your delicious 209-calorie Apple Pancake breakfast, you should also add 1 cup of skim milk (80 calories) and 3 slices of turkey bacon (90 calories) to round out the meal and raise it to the appropriate calorie level healthfully. Remember, the numbers in parentheses refer to the calorie counts of specific ingredients.

Confused? Don't be. All you have to do is follow the instructions in the "Make It a *Flat Belly Diet* Meal" boxes at the end of each recipe and you'll be assured of staying within the *Flat Belly Diet* rules, no matter which recipes you choose to try. Now let's get cookin'.

RECIPE INDEX

■ SEAFOOD pp. 198–209

Steamed Salmon with Snow Peas
Fish with Summer Squash
Roasted Fish with Artichokes
Grilled Salmon Steak
Lemony Stuffed Sole
Scallop Ceviche
Chai Scallops with Bok Choy
Sweet-and-Sour Shrimp
Sizzled Shrimp with Heirloom Tomatoes
Sesame Seared Scallops
Thai Sweet-Hot Shrimp
Seared Wild Salmon with Mango Salsa

■ MEAT pp. 210–214

Dijon Pork Chops with Cabbage
Mexican Pork Tenderloin
Stir-Fried Rice with Asian Vegetables
    and Beef
Vietnamese Beef Salad
Basic Balsamic Flank Steak

■ VEGETARIAN pp. 215–221

Broccoli and Tofu Stir-Fry with Toasted
    Almonds
Chickpea Salad
Zucchini Rotini
Stewed Vegetables
Stir-Fried Broccoli and Mushrooms
    with Tofu

Spaghetti Squash Casserole
Soybeans with Sesame and Scallions

■ SIDE DISHES pp. 222–228

Balsamic Roasted Carrots
Mini Sweet Potato Casseroles
Summer Squash Sauté
Wild Rice, Almond, and Cranberry Dressing
Guilt-Free Fries
Stir-Fried Asparagus with Ginger,
    Sesame, and Soy
Tuscan White Bean Spread

■ DESSERTS pp. 229–235

Plum and Nectarine Trifle
Chocolate Strawberries
Pumpkin-Maple Cheesecake
Oatmeal Cookies with Cranberries and
    Chocolate Chips
Chocolate Pudding with Bananas and
    Graham Crackers
Citrus Ricotta Cannoli
Double Chocolate Chip Oatmeal

Frittata with Smoked Salmon and Scallions

Preparation time: 10 minutes / Cooking time: 15 minutes /Makes 6 servings

2 teaspoons extra virgin olive oil

6 scallions (whites and 2″ of green), trimmed and coarsely chopped

6 egg whites

4 eggs

1½ teaspoons chopped fresh tarragon or ½ teaspoon dried

¼ cup cold water

½ teaspoon salt
Freshly ground black pepper

2 ounces thinly sliced smoked salmon, cut into ½″-wide pieces

MUFA: ¾ cup black olive tapenade

1. Preheat the oven to 350°F. Heat a heavy 8″ ovenproof skillet over medium heat for 1 minute. Add the olive oil and scallions and sauté, stirring, until soft.

2. In a medium bowl, whisk together the egg whites, eggs, tarragon, water, and salt. Season with pepper. Pour the mixture into the pan and lay salmon pieces on top. Cook, stirring periodically, for about 2 minutes, or until partially set.

3. Transfer to the oven and roast for about 6 to 8 minutes, or until firm, golden, and puffed. Remove. Use a spatula to release the frittata from the pan. Gently slide the frittata onto a warm serving platter. Spread 2 tablespoons of the tapenade on each plate, and place a slice of frittata on top.

■ **Eat One Serving:**

190

CALORIES,
10 g protein, 2 g carbohydrates, 15 g fat, 2.5 g saturated fat, 143 mg cholesterol, 537 mg sodium, 0 g fiber

MAKE IT A FLAT BELLY DIET MEAL
Serve with ½ cup frozen dark cherries, thawed (45), mixed into 1 cup nonfat plain Greek yogurt (112) and topped with 2 tablespoons toasted oats (37)

■ **TOTAL MEAL:**

384

CALORIES

Apple Pancakes

Preparation time: 20 minutes / Cooking time: 4 minutes / Makes 12 servings

²/₃ cup whole wheat flour

²/₃ cup unbleached all-purpose flour

¹/₃ cup cornmeal

1 tablespoon baking powder

1 teaspoon ground ginger

¹/₂ teaspoon baking soda

2 cups nonfat plain yogurt

³/₄ cup fat-free egg substitute

2 tablespoons canola oil

1 apple, peeled, cored, and coarsely grated

MUFA: 1¹/₂ cups pecans, chopped

1. In a large bowl, combine the flours, cornmeal, baking powder, ginger, baking soda, yogurt, egg substitute, and oil until combined.

2. Fold the grated apples into the batter.

3. Coat a large nonstick skillet with nonstick cooking spray and heat over medium heat.

4. For each pancake, spoon 2 to 3 tablespoons of the batter into the skillet. Cook for 2 minutes or until bubbles appear on the surface and edges set. Flip to the other side.

5. Cook until lightly browned, about 2 minutes. Repeat with the remaining batter.

6. Top each serving with 2 tablespoons of the chopped pecans.

■ **Eat One Serving:**

209

CALORIES,

6 g protein, 19 g carbohydrates, 13.5 g fat, 1 g saturated fat, 1 mg cholesterol, 208 mg sodium, 3 g fiber

MAKE IT A FLAT BELLY DIET MEAL

Serve with 1 cup skim milk (80) and 3 slices Applegate Farms® Organic Turkey Bacon (90)

■ **Total Meal:**

379

CALORIES

Nutty Fruit Muffins

Preparation time: 10 minutes / Cooking time: 20 minutes / Makes 12 servings

1¾ cups whole grain pastry flour

1½ teaspoons baking powder

1½ teaspoons ground cinnamon

½ teaspoon baking soda

¼ teaspoon salt

1 cup fat-free vanilla yogurt

½ cup brown sugar

1 egg

2 tablespoons canola oil

1 teaspoon vanilla extract

MUFA: 1½ cups walnuts, chopped

½ cup crushed pineapple in juice, drained

⅓ cup currants or raisins

¼ cup grated carrots

1. Preheat the oven to 400°F.

2. In a large bowl, combine first five ingredients. In a medium bowl, combine the yogurt, brown sugar, egg, oil, and vanilla extract. Stir the yogurt mixture into the flour mixture just until blended. (Lumps are okay.) Fold in the walnuts, pineapple, currants or raisins, and carrots.

3. Divide the batter evenly among 12 muffin cups coated with nonstick cooking spray.

4. Bake for 20 minutes, or until a toothpick inserted in the center of a muffin comes out clean.

5. Cool in pan on a wire rack for 5 minutes. Remove muffins from the pan to cool completely on the wire rack.

■ **Eat One Serving:**

242

CALORIES,

6 g protein, 29 g carbohydrates, 12.5 g fat, 1 g saturated fat, 18 mg cholesterol, 177 mg sodium, 3 g fiber

MAKE IT A FLAT BELLY DIET MEAL

Serve with 1 cup nonfat plain Greek yogurt (112)

■ **Total Meal:**

354

CALORIES

Pumpkin Spiced Oatmeal

Preparation and Cooking time: 2 minutes / Makes 1 serving

1 cup water
Pinch of salt
⅓ cup quick oats
¼ cup canned pure
pumpkin

MUFA: 2 tablespoons pecans, toasted and chopped

¼ teaspoon ground
cinnamon
2 teaspoons brown
sugar
Pinch of freshly grated
nutmeg
Pinch of ground cloves

1. In a saucepan over high heat, bring the water to a boil. Add the salt and oats. Cook, stirring, for 90 seconds.

2. Combine the remaining ingredients in a small bowl. Reduce the heat to low and stir in the pumpkin mixture.

■ **Eat One Serving:**

272

CALORIES,
6 g protein, 36 g carbohydrates, 13 g fat, 1 g saturated fat, 0 mg cholesterol, 305 mg sodium, 7 g fiber

MAKE IT A FLAT BELLY DIET MEAL
Serve with 1 cup skim milk (80)

■ **Total Meal:**

352

CALORIES

Southwestern Double-Corn and Pecan Muffins

Preparation time: 5 minutes / Cooking time: 18 minutes / Makes 12 servings

1 cup yellow cornmeal

1 cup whole grain pastry flour

¼ cup soy flour

2 teaspoons baking powder

¼ teaspoon ground cinnamon

⅛ teaspoon salt

1 egg

1 egg white

¾ cup skim milk

¼ cup canola oil

1½ cups frozen corn kernels

MUFA: 1½ cups pecans, chopped

½ cup golden raisins

1. Preheat the oven to 400°F.

2. In a large bowl, combine the cornmeal, pastry flour, soy flour, baking powder, cinnamon, and salt.

3. In a small bowl, combine the egg, egg white, milk, oil, corn, pecans, and raisins. Add the egg mixture to the flour mixture and stir just until blended. (Lumps are okay.) Fold in corn kernels, pecans, and raisins. Divide the batter evenly among 12 muffin cups coated with nonstick cooking spray.

4. Bake for 18 minutes, or until a toothpick inserted in the center of a muffin comes out clean. Cool in the pan on a wire rack for 5 minutes. Remove from the pan to cool completely on the wire rack.

■ **Eat One Serving:**

273

CALORIES,

6 g protein, 27 g carbohydrates, 17.5 g fat, 2 g saturated fat, 19 mg cholesterol, 113 mg sodium, 4 g fiber

MAKE IT A FLAT BELLY DIET MEAL

Serve with 1 cup skim milk (80)

■ **Total Meal:**

353

CALORIES

Fluted Egg Cups

Preparation time: 10 minutes / Cooking time: 5 minutes
Baking time: 20 minutes / Broiling time: 2 minutes / Makes 12 servings

6 large slices 100% whole wheat bread
2 tablespoons olive oil
1/3 cup chopped scallions
1 tablespoon chopped fresh basil
1 tablespoon chopped fresh Italian parsley
8 egg whites, lightly beaten
1/3 cup (about 1 1/2 ounces) shredded reduced-fat Cheddar cheese
1 tablespoon grated Parmesan cheese
1/2 teaspoon paprika

MUFA: 1 1/2 cups black olive tapenade

1. Preheat the oven to 350°F. With a rolling pin, slightly flatten the bread slices. Using a 3" round cookie cutter, cut 12 bread circles.

2. Coat a 12-cup mini-muffin pan with nonstick cooking spray. Line each cup with a bread round. Bake for 15 to 20 minutes, or until the edges are golden-brown.

3. Heat the oil in a large nonstick skillet over medium heat. Add the scallions, basil, and parsley; cook, stirring, for 1 to 2 minutes. Add the egg whites. Cook, stirring with a wooden spoon, for 1 to 2 minutes, or until almost set. Fold in the cheese and cook until the eggs are set.

4. Preheat the broiler. Spoon 1 tablespoon of the egg mixture into each bread cup and top with the Parmesan and paprika. Broil 4" from the heat source for 1 to 2 minutes, or until hot and lightly browned. Serve each cup with 2 tablespoons of the tapenade.

■ **Eat One Serving:**

172

CALORIES,
6 g protein, 6 g carbohydrates, 13 g fat, 2 g saturated fat, 3 mg cholesterol, 324 mg sodium, 1 g fiber

MAKE IT A FLAT BELLY DIET MEAL
Serve with 1/2 cup frozen dark cherries, thawed (45), mixed 1 cup nonfat Greek yogurt (112) and sprinkled with 2 tablespoons toasted oats (37)

■ **TOTAL MEAL:**

366

CALORIES

Fiesta Cornmeal Pudding

Preparation time: 10 minutes / Cooking time: 20 minutes
Baking time: 30 minutes / Makes 6 servings

2¼ cups water
½ teaspoon salt
¾ cup yellow cornmeal
1 tablespoon extra virgin olive oil
1 large red bell pepper, seeded and diced
4 scallions, chopped
2 large cloves garlic, minced

MUFA: 1½ cups pecans, chopped and divided

1 box (10 ounces) frozen chopped spinach, thawed and squeezed dry
1 large egg white
¼ teaspoon hot pepper sauce
½ cup (2 ounces) shredded sharp Cheddar cheese

1. Preheat the oven to 350°F.

2. Coat a 9″ baking dish with nonstick cooking spray.

3. In a large saucepan over high heat, bring the water to a boil. Add the salt. Reduce the heat to low. Whisk in the cornmeal in a slow, steady stream. Cover and cook, stirring frequently, for 10 minutes, or until very thick.

4. Meanwhile, heat the oil in a nonstick skillet over medium heat. Add the bell pepper; cook, stirring, for 4 minutes. Add the scallions and garlic; cook, stirring, for 2 minutes, or until the vegetables are tender. Add the bell pepper mixture, 1 cup of the pecans, spinach, egg white, and hot pepper sauce to the cornmeal. Stir to combine. Pour into the prepared baking dish. Sprinkle with the Cheddar.

5. Bake for 30 minutes, or until firm, puffed, and golden. Top with remaining pecans.

■ **Eat One Serving:**

344

CALORIES,
9 g protein, 21 g carbohydrates, 26 g fat, 3.5 g saturated fat, 7 mg cholesterol, 372 mg sodium, 4 g fiber

MAKE IT A FLAT BELLY DIET MEAL
Serve with 2 slices Applegate Farms® Organic Bacon (60)

■ **TOTAL MEAL:**

404

CALORIES

Grilled Portobello and Roasted Pepper Burgers

Preparation time: 4 minutes / Cooking time: 6 minutes / Makes 2 servings

4 small portobello mushroom caps (8 ounces total), stems removed

4 teaspoons balsamic vinegar

2 jarred, roasted red bell pepper halves

2 100% whole wheat buns

MUFA: 2 tablespoons prepared pesto

4 leaves frisée lettuce

1. Preheat a grill pan over medium heat.

2. Grill the mushrooms for 8 minutes, turning halfway during cooking and brushing with the vinegar. Warm the pepper halves and buns on the grill pan.

3. Spread 1 tablespoon pesto on each bun bottom, then place 2 mushrooms and 1 pepper slice on each bun bottom, adding 2 pieces of frisée to each. Drizzle with additional vinegar, if desired, and cap with bun top.

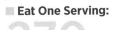

■ **Eat One Serving:**

270

CALORIES,
10 g protein, 37 g carbohydrates, 9.5 g fat, 2.5 g saturated fat, 5 mg cholesterol, 614 mg sodium, 5 g fiber

MAKE IT A FLAT BELLY DIET MEAL
Add a dessert: Mix ¼ cup nonfat ricotta cheese (50) with 1 teaspoon honey (21) and top with ½ cup pear slices (50)

■ **TOTAL MEAL:**

391

CALORIES

Wasabi Salmon Sandwiches

Preparation time: 8 minutes / Makes 4 servings

¼ cup fat-free mayonnaise

¼–½ teaspoon wasabi paste

2 cups (about 8 ounces) canned Alaskan wild salmon

8 thin slices 100% whole wheat bread, toasted

4 thin slices red onion

4 thin rings red bell pepper

MUFA: 1 cup sliced avocado

¼ cup sliced pickled ginger

1 cup arugula

1. In a small bowl, combine the mayonnaise and wasabi paste until smooth. Start with ¼ teaspoon of the paste and add more to suit your taste. Gently fold in the salmon.

2. Place 4 slices of the bread on a flat surface and top each with ½ cup of the salmon mixture, 1 onion slice separated into rings, 1 pepper ring, ¼ cup avocado, 1 tablespoon ginger, and ¼ cup arugula. Top with the remaining 4 slices of bread.

■ **Eat One Serving:**

243

CALORIES,

12 g protein, 26 g carbohydrates, 10 g fat, 1.5 g saturated fat, 21 mg cholesterol, 355 mg sodium, 6 g fiber

MAKE IT A FLAT BELLY DIET MEAL

Serve with ⅔ cup frozen, thawed Cascadian Farm® Organic Edamame (120)

■ **TOTAL MEAL:**

363

CALORIES

Tuna Bruschetta

Preparation time: 5 minutes / Makes 2 servings

1 can (6 ounces)
reduced-sodium
water-packed tuna,
drained and flaked
1 cup canned
no-salt-added, diced
tomatoes, drained
¼ cup (1 ounce)
crumbled reduced-fat
feta cheese

**MUFA: ¼ cup black olive
tapenade**

1 tablespoon lemon juice
4 slices 100% whole
wheat bread, toasted

1. In a bowl, combine the
tuna, tomatoes, feta, and
lemon juice.

2. Spread the tapenade
over 2 slices of the toast
and top each with half of
the tuna mixture. Top with
the remaining 2 slices of
toast.

■ **Eat One Serving:**

391

CALORIES,
35 g protein, 30 g
carbohydrates,
14.5 g fat, 2.5 g
saturated fat,
43 mg cholesterol,
717 mg sodium,
6 g fiber

**A SINGLE SERVING
OF THIS RECIPE
COUNTS AS A FLAT
BELLY DIET MEAL
WITHOUT ANY
ADD-ONS!**

Fresh Pea Soup with Mint

Preparation time: 7 minutes / Cooking time: 15 minutes
Chilling time: 1 hour / Makes 4 servings

1 tablespoon olive oil

2 scallions, green parts only, cut into 4" pieces

1 rib celery, trimmed and cut into 2" pieces

½ medium onion, finely chopped

3 cups low-sodium chicken or vegetable broth

4 cups peas, fresh, or frozen and thawed

¼ teaspoon salt

⅓ cup fresh mint leaves

½ cup nonfat plain Greek yogurt

MUFA: ½ cup pumpkin seeds, toasted

1. Heat the oil in a large saucepan over medium-high heat. Add the scallions, celery, and onion. Cook, stirring, for about 5 minutes, or until the vegetables are tender.

2. Add the broth and bring to a boil. Add the peas and salt. Simmer for 10 minutes.

3. Carefully transfer the mixture to the bowl of a food processor fitted with a metal blade or into a blender (in batches, if necessary). Add the mint. Puree until smooth. Cover and chill for at least 1 hour.

4. Spoon the soup into 4 serving bowls. Dollop 2 tablespoons of yogurt in the center of each and sprinkle with 2 tablespoons of the pumpkin seeds.

■ **Eat One Serving:**

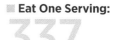

CALORIES,

23 g protein, 29 g carbohydrates, 16.5 g fat, 3 g saturated fat, 4 mg cholesterol, 439 mg sodium, 8 g fiber

MAKE IT A FLAT BELLY DIET MEAL

Serve with 1 cup grapes (60)

■ **TOTAL MEAL:**

397

CALORIES

Asian Soup
with Shrimp Dumplings

Preparation time: 15 minutes / Cooking time: 15 minutes / Makes 4 servings

4 cloves garlic, smashed, divided

½" piece fresh ginger, peeled and smashed, divided

½ pound medium shrimp, peeled and deveined

¼ cup fresh cilantro

2 teaspoons cornstarch

2 tablespoons water

1 tablespoon reduced-sodium soy sauce

½ teaspoon toasted sesame oil

6 cups low-sodium chicken broth

1 stalk lemongrass, cut in half and smashed

½ teaspoon red pepper flakes

1 cup cooked kale

MUFA: ½ cup dry-roasted peanuts, chopped

1. In a food processor, mince half of the garlic and ginger. Add the shrimp and cilantro; pulse to combine. In a small bowl, whisk together the cornstarch and water until the cornstarch is dissolved. Add to the food processor along with the soy sauce and oil. Pulse to combine. Set aside.

2. In a large saucepan over high heat, bring to a boil the broth, lemongrass, red pepper flakes, and the remaining garlic and ginger. Reduce the heat to low and let simmer.

3. Meanwhile, moisten your clean hands and roll the shrimp mixture into 12 balls. Drop the shrimp dumplings one at a time into the simmering soup. Cook for 6 minutes or until opaque. Remove and discard the lemongrass. Divide the greens evenly among 4 serving bowls and ladle the soup and 3 dumplings on top of each. Sprinkle with 2 tablespoons of the peanuts.

■ **Eat One Serving:**

252

CALORIES,
24 g protein, 13 g carbohydrates, 13 g fat, 2 g saturated fat, 86 mg cholesterol, 335 mg sodium, 2 g fiber

MAKE IT A FLAT BELLY DIET MEAL
Serve with 1 cup red pepper slices (40) and ¼ cup hummus for dipping (100)

■ **TOTAL MEAL:**

392

CALORIES

Mexican Chicken Soup

Preparation time: 4 minutes / Cooking time: 16 minutes / Makes 4 servings

5 cups low-sodium chicken broth

5 white corn tortillas (6"), sliced into ¼" strips

12 ounces boneless, skinless chicken breast, thinly sliced crosswise

½ canned chipotle chile pepper, sliced, or 2 tablespoons hot salsa

¾ cup halved grape tomatoes

MUFA: 1 cup chopped avocado

¼ cup fresh cilantro leaves

1. In a large heavy saucepan, bring the broth to a boil, covered over high heat.

2. Meanwhile, scatter the tortilla strips on a toaster oven tray. Toast, turning the strips occasionally, until golden-brown in spots, about 5 minutes. Remove the tray from toaster oven and set the tortilla strips aside.

3. When the broth boils, add the chicken, chile pepper, and tomatoes and return to a boil. Remove from the heat. Divide the tortilla strips, avocado, and cilantro leaves evenly among 4 bowls, mounding them in the center. Ladle the soup into bowls.

■ **Eat One Serving:**

282

CALORIES,
29 g protein, 24 g carbohydrates, 9.5 g fat, 1.5 g saturated fat, 49 mg cholesterol, 153 mg sodium, 5 g fiber

MAKE IT A FLAT BELLY DIET MEAL
Serve with 2 cups baby greens (10) tossed with 2 tablespoons Newman's Own® Light Balsamic Vinaigrette (45) and 1 cup of grapes (60)

■ **TOTAL MEAL:**

397

CALORIES

Slow Cooker Chili

Preparation time: 10 minutes / Cooking time: 4 to 6 hours / Makes 4 servings

1 can (28 ounces) salt-free whole tomatoes

1 medium green bell pepper, seeded and chopped

1 can (14 ounces) chili beans, rinsed and drained

½ package (12 ounces) fat-free soy crumbles

Chili powder

1 tablespoon minced onion

1 tablespoon olive oil

MUFA: 1 cup chopped avocado

1. In a 4-quart slow cooker, combine the whole tomatoes, pepper, beans, soy crumbles, chili powder to taste, onion, and oil. Cover and cook on high setting for 4 to 6 hours or on medium setting for 8 hours, or until thick. Garnish each serving with ¼ cup of the avocado.

■ **Eat One Serving:**

358

CALORIES,
24 g protein,
34 g carbohydrates,
13.5 g fat, 2 g saturated fat, 0 mg cholesterol, 570 mg sodium, 13 g fiber

A SINGLE SERVING OF THIS RECIPE COUNTS AS A FLAT BELLY DIET MEAL WITHOUT ANY ADD-ONS!

Black Bean Chili

Preparation time: 5 minutes / Cooking time: 3 minutes / Makes 2 servings

1 cup fat-free soy
  crumbles
1 cup canned,
  no-salt-added black
  beans, rinsed and
  drained
1 cup lower-sodium
  chipotle-flavored salsa
2 teaspoons chili powder
1 teaspoon ground
  cumin

**MUFA: ½ cup mashed
  avocado**

1. In a saucepan over
medium heat, combine the
soy crumbles, beans, salsa,
chili powder, and cumin.
Cook, stirring occasionally,
for about 3 minutes, or
until heated through. Top
each serving with ¼ cup of
the avocado.

■ **Eat One Serving:**

338

CALORIES,
20 g protein, 39 g
carbohydrates,
9 g fat, 1.7 g
saturated fat, 0 mg
cholesterol, 674 mg
sodium, 15 g fiber

**MAKE IT A FLAT
BELLY DIET MEAL**
Serve with 1 cup
sliced red bell
pepper (40)

■ **TOTAL MEAL:**

378

CALORIES

Hearty Country Vegetable Soup

Preparation time: 15 minutes / Cooking time: 2 hours 15 minutes
Makes 8 servings

MUFA: ½ cup olive oil, divided

½ large onion, chopped
3 ribs celery, chopped
1 small head green cabbage, chopped
2 carrots, chopped
2 cloves garlic, minced
½ cup dried white beans
3 cans (14.5 ounces each) low-sodium vegetable broth
1½ teaspoons chopped fresh thyme, or ½ teaspoon dried
1½ teaspoons chopped fresh savory or sage, or ½ teaspoon dried
½ pound green beans, cut into 1" pieces
1 zucchini, halved lengthwise and sliced

1. Heat ¼ cup oil in a soup pot over medium-low heat. Stir in the onion, celery, cabbage, carrots, and garlic. Cover and cook for 12 to 15 minutes, stirring occasionally. Add the beans and 5 cups of the broth. Bring the mixture to a boil. Reduce the heat to medium-low and stir in the thyme and savory. Cover and cook for 1 to 1½ hours, or until the beans are almost tender, adding some of the remaining broth if the soup becomes too thick.

2. Stir in the green beans and zucchini. Partially cover and cook for 20 to 30 minutes, or until the green beans are tender. Divide among 8 bowls. Drizzle ½ tablespoon of the remaining oil in each bowl.

■ **Eat One Serving:**

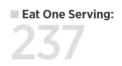

237

CALORIES,
6 g protein, 23 g carbohydrates, 14 g fat, 2 g saturated fat, 0 mg cholesterol, 353 mg sodium, 7 g fiber

MAKE IT A FLAT BELLY DIET MEAL
Serve with 2 cups baby greens (15) and 1 cup halved grape tomatoes (30) tossed with 2 tablespoons Annie's Naturals® Goddess Dressing (90)

■ **TOTAL MEAL:**

372

CALORIES

Turnip and Carrot Soup with Parmesan

Preparation time: 15 minutes / Cooking time: 20 minutes / Makes 8 servings

1 pound white turnips, peeled and quartered

4 large carrots, cut into chunks

2 large red or white new potatoes, quartered

1 large onion, chopped

5 cloves garlic, smashed

1½ cups low-sodium chicken broth

1½ cups water

1½ teaspoons chopped fresh thyme, or ½ teaspoon dried

1½ teaspoons chopped fresh sage, or ½ teaspoon dried

¼ teaspoon salt

¼ teaspoon freshly ground black pepper

1 cup 1% milk

½ cup (2 ounces) grated Parmesan cheese

MUFA: 1 cup pine nuts, toasted

1. In a large saucepan or Dutch oven, combine the turnips, carrots, potatoes, onion, garlic, broth, water, thyme, sage, salt, and pepper. Bring to a boil over high heat. Reduce the heat to medium, cover, and simmer for 20 minutes, or until the vegetables are very tender.

2. In batches, transfer the cooked vegetables into the bowl of a food processor fitted with a metal blade or into a blender, and puree until smooth. When all the soup has been pureed, return it to the pan. Stir in the milk. Cook over low heat just until heated through (do not boil). Remove from the heat and stir in the Parmesan. Ladle into bowls and top each with 2 tablespoons of the pine nuts.

■ **Eat One Serving:**

261

CALORIES,
9 g protein, 28 g carbohydrates, 13.5 g fat, 2 g saturated fat, 7 mg cholesterol, 263 mg sodium, 5 g fiber

MAKE IT A FLAT BELLY DIET MEAL
Serve with 2 Laughing Cow® Light Garlic & Herb Cheese wedges (70) and 2 Ry Krisp® crackers (70)

■ **TOTAL MEAL:**

401

CALORIES

Chilled Strawberry Soup

Preparation time: 5 minutes / Cooking time: 4 minutes /
Cooling time: 5 minutes / Chilling time: 60 minutes / Makes 4 servings

2 cups fresh
strawberries, hulled

¾ cup white grape juice

¼ cup orange juice

¼ teaspoon lemon
extract

⅛ teaspoon freshly
grated nutmeg

1 cup fat-free vanilla
yogurt

**MUFA: ½ cup slivered
almonds, toasted**

1. In a 2-quart saucepan,
bring the strawberries,
grape juice, orange juice,
lemon extract, and nutmeg
to a boil over medium
heat, stirring occasionally.
Reduce the heat and
simmer for 1 minute.
Remove from the heat and
allow to cool for 5 minutes.

2. Transfer the soup to a
blender and puree until
smooth. Pour into a large
bowl. Chill for 30 minutes.
Whisk in the yogurt and
chill another 30 minutes
before serving. Divide
evenly into 4 bowls, and top
each with 2 tablespoons of
the almonds.

■ **Eat One Serving:**

195

CALORIES,
7 g protein, 28 g
carbohydrates,
7 g fat, 0.5 g
saturated fat, 1 mg
cholesterol, 48 mg
sodium, 3 g fiber

**MAKE IT A FLAT
BELLY DIET MEAL**
Serve with
5 Ry Krisp®
crackers (175)

■ **TOTAL MEAL:**

370

CALORIES

Cucumber and Melon Salad with Watercress, Herbs, and Feta

Preparation time: 25 minutes / Makes 4 servings

DRESSING

2 teaspoons extra virgin olive oil

2 tablespoons freshly squeezed lemon juice

2 tablespoons white wine vinegar

1 tablespoon minced shallot

1 teaspoon sugar

½ teaspoon salt

½ teaspoon freshly ground black pepper

SALAD

3 cucumbers, peeled and chopped (about 6 cups)

8 cups melon balls (such as 1 honeydew or various types)

1 bunch watercress, large stems discarded

½ cup fresh mint leaves

½ cup crumbled feta cheese

MUFA: ½ cup pine nuts, toasted

1 tablespoon chopped kalamata olives

1. To prepare the dressing: In a small bowl, whisk together the oil, lemon juice, vinegar, shallot, sugar, salt, and pepper.

2. To prepare the salad: In a large bowl, combine the cucumbers, melon balls, watercress, mint, feta, pine nuts, and olives. Pour the dressing on the salad and toss gently to coat.

■ **Eat One Serving:**

354

CALORIES,

9 g protein, 43 g carbohydrates, 19 g fat, 4 g saturated fat, 17 mg cholesterol, 548 mg sodium, 5 g fiber

A SINGLE SERVING OF THIS RECIPE COUNTS AS A FLAT BELLY DIET MEAL WITHOUT ANY ADD-ONS!

Carrot-Walnut Salad

Preparation time: 20 minutes / Makes 4 servings

⅓ cup golden raisins

2 tablespoons rice wine vinegar

1 tablespoon canola oil

2 teaspoons freshly squeezed lemon juice (about 1 lemon)

1 teaspoon honey

⅛ teaspoon salt

4 large carrots, grated

MUFA: ½ cup walnuts, toasted and chopped

¼ cup chopped fresh Italian parsley

1. Soak the raisins in hot water for 20 minutes to plump them. Drain.

2. In a small bowl, whisk together the vinegar, oil, lemon juice, honey, and salt.

3. Combine the carrots, walnuts, parsley, raisins, and dressing in a medium bowl and toss to coat. Divide evenly among 4 salad plates.

■ **Eat One Serving:**

199

CALORIES,

3 g protein, 20 g carbohydrates, 13.5 g fat, 1.5 g saturated fat, 0 mg cholesterol, 127 mg sodium, 4 g fiber

MAKE IT A FLAT BELLY DIET MEAL

Serve with 1 slice Food for Life® Ezekiel 4:9® Sesame Sprouted Bread (80) and 1 apple (80)

■ **TOTAL MEAL:**

359

CALORIES

Sugar Snap Pea and Fennel Salad with Apple Cider Vinaigrette

Preparation time: 15 minutes / Makes 6 servings

2 tablespoons apple cider vinegar

2 teaspoons honey

1½ teaspoons extra virgin olive oil

¾ teaspoon Dijon mustard

¼ teaspoon salt

2½ cups sugar snap peas, tough strings removed

1½ cups shelled fresh peas

1 small fennel bulb, trimmed, halved, and cut into bite-size strips

¼ cup grated sweet onion

1 tablespoon chopped fresh tarragon

2 teaspoons finely chopped shallots
Freshly ground black pepper

MUFA: ¾ cup sunflower seeds

1. Whisk together the vinegar, honey, oil, mustard, and salt in a large bowl. Add the snap peas, peas, fennel, onion, tarragon, and shallot. Toss to coat and season to taste with pepper. Divide evenly among 6 salad plates and sprinkle with the sunflower seeds.

■ **Eat One Serving:**

189

CALORIES,
8 g protein, 19 g carbohydrates, 10.5 g fat, 1 g saturated fat, 0 mg cholesterol, 141 mg sodium, 6 g fiber

MAKE IT A FLAT BELLY DIET MEAL
Serve with ½ cup canned Alaskan wild salmon (180)

■ **TOTAL MEAL:**

369

CALORIES

Crab Salad with Avocado and Pomelo

Preparation time: 22 minutes / Makes 4 servings

DRESSING

2 tablespoons orange juice

2 teaspoons extra virgin olive oil

2 tablespoons white wine vinegar

2 teaspoons finely chopped fresh tarragon or chervil

½ teaspoon freshly grated orange zest

½ teaspoon salt

¼ teaspoon dry mustard

¼ teaspoon freshly ground black pepper

SALAD

2 heads butterhead lettuce, separated into leaves (about 8 cups)

2 medium sweet onions (such as Vidalia), sliced (about 2 cups)

2 pomelos, peeled and cut into sections (about 4 cups) (see Note)

MUFA: 1 cup sliced avocado

1 cup lump crabmeat

1 tablespoon chopped blanched hazelnuts, toasted

1. To prepare the dressing: In a medium bowl, whisk together the orange juice, oil, vinegar, tarragon or chervil, orange zest, salt, mustard, and pepper.

2. To prepare the salad: In a large bowl, combine the lettuce, onions, and pomelo. Add the dressing and toss to coat. Mound the salad evenly among 4 plates. Top with avocado slices, ¼ cup of the crabmeat, and hazelnuts.

Note: Replace the pomelos with grapefruit if they're not available.

■ **Eat One Serving:**

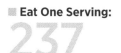

CALORIES,
11 g protein, 31 g carbohydrates, 10 g fat, 1.5 g saturated fat, 30 mg cholesterol, 335 mg sodium, 7 g fiber

MAKE IT A FLAT BELLY DIET MEAL
Serve with 4 Ry Krisp® crackers (140)

■ **TOTAL MEAL:**

377

CALORIES

Curried Barley and Shrimp Salad

Preparation time: 20 minutes / Cooking time: 45 minutes / Makes 6 servings

3 cups water
1 teaspoon curry powder
½ teaspoon turmeric
1 cup barley
¼ cup plus 1 tablespoon freshly squeezed lime juice (about 4 limes)
1 tablespoon vegetable oil
2 teaspoons finely chopped jalapeño chile pepper, seeded (see Note)
1 clove garlic, minced
¼ teaspoon salt
1 pound small cooked shrimp, peeled and deveined
1½ cups seeded and diced tomatoes
½ cup chopped green bell pepper
½ cup chopped peeled cucumber
12 cups baby greens
¼ cup chopped fresh basil

MUFA: ¾ cup pumpkin seeds, toasted

1. In a large saucepan over high heat, bring the water, curry, and turmeric to a boil. Stir in the barley. Cover and reduce the heat to low. Cook for about 45 minutes, or until the water is absorbed and the barley is tender. Remove from heat. Meanwhile, in a large bowl, whisk together the lime juice, oil, chile pepper, garlic, and salt. Add the shrimp, tomatoes, bell pepper, cucumber, and barley. Toss to coat.

2. Spoon the salad on top of 2 cups of baby greens per plate. Divide salad evenly and sprinkle with the basil and the pumpkin seeds.

Note: Wear plastic gloves and keep hands away from eyes when handling fresh chile peppers.

■ **Eat One Serving:**

338

CALORIES,
24 g protein, 35 g carbohydrates, 12.5 g fat, 2.5 g saturated fat, 115 mg cholesterol, 273 mg sodium, 7 g fiber

MAKE IT A FLAT BELLY DIET MEAL
Serve on a bed of 2 cups baby greens (15)

■ **TOTAL MEAL:**

353

CALORIES

Beet and Goat Cheese Salad

Preparation time: 25 minutes / Makes 6 servings

SALAD
- 6 cups baby greens
- 8 medium canned beets (about 8 ounces), drained and sliced

MUFA: ¾ cup toasted walnut halves

DRESSING
- 2 teaspoons olive oil
- 3 tablespoons white wine vinegar
- ¼ teaspoon salt
  Freshly ground black pepper
- 2 ounces soft goat cheese, crumbled

1. To prepare the salad: Combine the greens, beets, and walnuts in a large bowl.

2. To prepare the dressing: Pour the olive oil into a small bowl and gradually whisk in the vinegar and salt. Season to taste with pepper. Pour over the salad and toss gently. Divide evenly among 6 plates and sprinkle with the cheese.

■ Eat One Serving:

147

CALORIES,
5 g protein, 6 g carbohydrates, 12.5 g fat, 3 g saturated fat, 7 mg cholesterol, 227 mg sodium, 2 g fiber

MAKE IT A FLAT BELLY DIET MEAL
Serve with 1 Thomas'® Multigrain Pita (140) and ¼ cup hummus (100)

■ TOTAL MEAL:

387

CALORIES

Warm Quinoa Salad

Preparation time: 8 minutes / Cooking time: 10 minutes / Makes 4 servings

2 cups water

1 cup quinoa, rinsed and drained

1 cup chopped radicchio (about ½ head), plus leaves for garnish

½ cup chopped fresh cilantro

½ cup golden raisins

½ cup fat-free honey mustard dressing

½ teaspoon salt
Freshly ground black pepper

MUFA: ½ cup cashews, toasted and chopped

1. In a medium saucepan, over high heat, bring the water and quinoa to a boil. Reduce the heat to a simmer, cover, and cook for about 5 minutes, or until all the liquid is absorbed.

2. Transfer the quinoa to a medium serving bowl. Add the chopped radicchio, cilantro, raisins, dressing, and salt. Toss to coat. Season to taste with pepper. Place the radicchio leaves onto 4 plates, divide the salad evenly, and sprinkle each with 2 table-spoons of the cashews.

■ **Eat One Serving:**

363

CALORIES,
9 g protein, 60 g carbohydrates, 10.5 g fat, 2 g saturated fat, 0 mg cholesterol, 435 mg sodium, 4g fiber

A SINGLE SERVING OF THIS RECIPE COUNTS AS A FLAT BELLY DIET MEAL WITHOUT ANY ADD-ONS!

Italian Shrimp and Pasta Salad

Preparation time: 7 minutes / Cooking time: 10 minutes / Makes 2 servings

½ cup whole wheat fusilli pasta
1 can (3 ounces) tiny shrimp, drained
½ cup halved grape tomatoes
¼ cup torn fresh basil
1 teaspoon Italian seasoning
1 teaspoon olive oil

MUFA: ¼ cup pine nuts, toasted

1. In a medium pot of rapidly boiling water, cook the pasta for 8 to 10 minutes, or until al dente. Drain and rinse with cold water until cool to the touch.

2. In a large bowl, combine the shrimp, tomatoes, basil, Italian seasoning, oil, and pasta. Toss to coat and sprinkle with the nuts.

■ **Eat One Serving:**

231

CALORIES,
12 g protein, 15 g carbohydrates, 15 g fat, 1 g saturated fat, 87 mg cholesterol, 362 mg sodium, 3 g fiber

MAKE IT A FLAT BELLY DIET MEAL
Serve with 1 string cheese (80) and 1 cup grapes (60)

■ **TOTAL MEAL:**

371

CALORIES

Turkey-Avocado Cobb Salad

Preparation time: 8 minutes / Cooking time: 7 minutes / Makes 4 servings

1 pound turkey breast cutlets

2 teaspoons olive oil, plus 1 teaspoon for the turkey

2 tablespoons cider vinegar

1 tablespoon water

1 teaspoon Dijon mustard

8 cups baby spinach

4 slices cooked turkey bacon, chopped

MUFA: 1 cup diced avocado

4 cherry tomatoes, halved

1 ounce blue cheese, crumbled
Freshly ground black pepper

1. Preheat a grill pan on medium-high heat for 2 minutes. Brush the turkey with 1 teaspoon of the oil. Grill the turkey for 4 minutes, flip, and continue cooking for about 3 minutes longer, or until no longer pink. Cut into chunks.

2. In a glass jar, combine the vinegar, water, mustard, and the remaining 2 teaspoons oil. Cover and shake well.

3. In a large bowl, combine the spinach with 2 tablespoons of the dressing. Toss to coat the leaves. Arrange the turkey, bacon, avocados, tomatoes, and cheese over the spinach. Drizzle on the remaining dressing, and season with pepper to taste.

■ Eat One Serving:

288

CALORIES,

34 g protein, 10 g carbohydrates, 13.5 g fat, 3.1 g saturated fat, 57 mg cholesterol, 473 mg sodium, 5 g fiber

MAKE IT A FLAT BELLY DIET MEAL
Serve with 1 medium apple (80)

■ TOTAL MEAL:

368

CALORIES

Soba Noodle Salad with Snow Peas

Preparation time: 15 minutes / Makes 6 servings

8 ounces dry soba noodles or whole wheat spaghetti

2 tablespoons honey

2 tablespoons freshly squeezed lime juice (about 2 limes)

2 tablespoons rice wine vinegar

2 tablespoons reduced-sodium soy sauce

1 tablespoon grated fresh ginger

1/4 teaspoon red pepper flakes

2 tablespoons peanut oil

2 cups shredded cooked chicken

2 cups julienned fresh snow peas

2 red bell peppers, seeded and thinly sliced lengthwise

1 cup grated carrots

MUFA: 1½ cups diced avocado

1/4 cup fresh cilantro, coarsely chopped

1. Cook the noodles according to the package directions. Drain and rinse with cold water. Set aside.

2. In a large bowl, whisk together the honey, lime juice, vinegar, soy sauce, ginger, and pepper flakes. Whisk in the oil in a steady stream.

3. Fold in the chicken, snow peas, bell peppers, carrots, avocado, cilantro, and noodles.

■ **Eat One Serving:**

352

CALORIES,
20 g protein, 48 g carbohydrates, 11 g fat, 2 g saturated fat, 26 mg cholesterol, 392 mg sodium, 6 g fiber

A SINGLE SERVING OF THIS RECIPE COUNTS AS A FLAT BELLY DIET MEAL WITHOUT ANY ADD-ONS!

Spinach Salad

Preparation time: 8 minutes / Makes 1 serving

2 tablespoons balsamic vinegar

MUFA: 1 tablespoon olive oil

⅛ teaspoon freshly ground black pepper

3 cups fresh baby spinach leaves

¼ cup sliced mushrooms

¼ cup halved yellow grape tomatoes

1 small red bell pepper, seeded and sliced into strips

1. In a salad or pasta bowl, whisk together the vinegar, oil, and black pepper. Add the spinach and toss to coat. Top with the mushrooms, tomatoes, and bell pepper.

■ **Eat One Serving:**

209

CALORIES,
4 g protein, 20 g carbohydrates, 14 g fat, 2 g saturated fat, 0 mg cholesterol, 353 mg sodium, 6 g fiber

MAKE IT A FLAT BELLY DIET MEAL
Serve with 4 Ry Krisp® crackers (105) and 2 Laughing Cow® Light Garlic & Herb wedges (70)

■ **TOTAL MEAL:**

384

CALORIES

Herb and Mesclun Salad with Grilled Shrimp

Preparation time: 30 minutes / Marinating time: 20 minutes
Cooking time: 4 minutes / Makes 4 servings

¼ cup fresh lime juice, divided (about 4 limes)

½ teaspoon ground cumin, divided

¼ teaspoon salt, divided

¼ teaspoon red pepper flakes, divided

1 pound large shrimp, peeled and deveined

6 cups mixed baby greens

1 cup fresh mint

1 cup fresh cilantro

1 cup fresh flat-leaf parsley

1 small red onion, thinly sliced

2 tablespoons vegetable oil

MUFA: ½ cup slivered almonds, toasted

1. In medium bowl, whisk together 2 tablespoons of the lime juice, ¼ teaspoon of the cumin, ⅛ teaspoon of the salt, and a pinch of the pepper flakes. Stir in the shrimp and chill for 20 minutes.

2. Meanwhile, in a serving bowl, toss together the baby greens, mint, cilantro, parsley, and onion. Chill until ready to serve.

3. In a small bowl, whisk together the oil, ¼ teaspoon cumin, ⅛ teaspoon salt, the remaining pepper flakes, and 2 tablespoons of the lime juice.

4. Grill or broil the shrimp for about 2 minutes each side, or until just opaque. Add the shrimp and dressing to the greens. Toss gently to coat. Divide evenly among 4 plates and top with the almonds.

■ Eat One Serving:

280

CALORIES,
25 g protein, 11 g carbohydrates, 16 g fat, 1.5 g saturated fat, 151 mg cholesterol, 327 mg sodium, 5 g fiber

MAKE IT A FLAT BELLY DIET MEAL
Serve with ½ Thomas'® Multigrain Sahara Pita (70) and 2 tablespoons hummus (50)

■ TOTAL MEAL:

400

CALORIES

Curried Potato Salad

Preparation time: 10 minutes / Makes 4 servings

1 pound potatoes, boiled and cubed

2 scallions, chopped

MUFA: ½ cup sliced almonds, toasted

¼ cup raisins

½ cup fat-free plain yogurt

2 tablespoons mango chutney

2 teaspoons curry powder

1. Place the potatoes in a large bowl and stir in the scallions, almonds, and raisins.

2. In a small bowl, whisk together the yogurt, chutney, and curry powder. Pour over the potatoes and toss to combine well. Divide evenly among 4 plates and serve.

■ **Eat One Serving:**

226

CALORIES,
6 g protein, 39 g carbohydrates, 6.5 g fat, 0.5 g saturated fat, 1 mg cholesterol, 26 mg sodium, 4 g dietary fiber

MAKE IT A FLAT BELLY DIET MEAL
Serve on a bed of 2 cups baby greens (15) with 3 ounces grilled chicken breast (90) and 1 medium apple (80)

■ **TOTAL MEAL:**

411

CALORIES

Bitter Greens with Hot Vinaigrette Dressing

Preparation time: 5 minutes / Cooking time: 7 minutes / Makes 4 servings

½ cup balsamic vinegar

2 teaspoons honey

1 teaspoon Dijon mustard

2 cloves garlic, minced

1½ teaspoons chopped fresh tarragon, or ½ teaspoon dried

⅛ teaspoon freshly ground black pepper

4 cups torn bitter greens, such as dandelion

2 slices turkey bacon, cooked until crisp and crumbled

MUFA: ½ cup pine nuts, toasted

1. Arrange the greens on 4 salad plates.

2. In a 1-quart saucepan, whisk together the vinegar, honey, mustard, garlic, tarragon, and pepper. Cook over medium heat for 1 to 2 minutes, or until the mixture is hot but not boiling.

3. Spoon immediately over the greens and toss well to coat. Sprinkle each salad evenly with bacon and pine nuts.

■ **Eat One Serving:**

198

CALORIES,

5 g protein, 18 g carbohydrates, 13 g fat, 2 g saturated fat, 8 mg cholesterol, 141 mg sodium, 2 g fiber

MAKE IT A FLAT BELLY DIET MEAL

Serve with 3 ounces grilled pork tenderloin (115) and ¼ cup steamed brown rice (55)

■ **TOTAL MEAL:**

368

CALORIES

Moroccan Carrot Salad with Toasted Cumin

Preparation time: 10 minutes / Cooking time: 2 minutes / Makes 4 servings

¾ teaspoon ground cumin

¼ teaspoon ground coriander

½ cup reduced-fat sour cream

MUFA: ¼ cup organic cold-pressed flaxseed oil

1 tablespoon plus 1 teaspoon lemon juice (about 1 lemon)

1½ teaspoons extra virgin olive oil

¼ teaspoon freshly grated orange zest

¼ teaspoon salt

7 medium carrots, peeled and grated

½ cup currants

2 tablespoons finely chopped red onion

1. In a small dry skillet over medium heat, toast the cumin and coriander, stirring often, for 2 minutes, or until fragrant and slightly darker in color. Place in a medium bowl and let cool. Stir in the sour cream, flaxseed oil, lemon juice, olive oil, orange zest, and salt.

2. Add the carrots, currants, and onion, and toss to coat well. Divide evenly among 4 plates.

■ **Eat One Serving:**

276

CALORIES,
3 g protein, 26 g carbohydrates, 19.5 g fat, 4 g saturated fat, 12 mg cholesterol, 234 mg sodium, 4 g fiber

MAKE IT A FLAT BELLY DIET MEAL

Serve with 3 ounces broiled medium shrimp (90)

■ **TOTAL MEAL:**

366

CALORIES

Spinach Salad with Radishes and Walnuts

Preparation time: 10 minutes / Makes 4 servings

1 tablespoon freshly squeezed lemon juice (about 1 lemon)

2 teaspoons white wine vinegar

Salt

Freshly ground black pepper

¼ cup extra virgin olive oil

5 ounces baby spinach leaves

4 medium radishes, thinly sliced

MUFA: ½ cup walnut halves

1. In a large bowl, whisk together the lemon juice and vinegar. Season to taste with salt and pepper. Whisk in the olive oil slowly.

2. When ready to serve, toss together the spinach and radishes and toss with the dressing to coat. Divide evenly among 4 salad plates and sprinkle each with 2 tablespoons of the walnuts.

■ **Eat One Serving:**

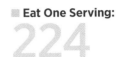

CALORIES,
3 g protein, 6 g carbohydrates, 22 g fat, 2.5 g saturated fat, 0 mg cholesterol, 204 mg sodium, 3 g fiber

MAKE IT A FLAT BELLY DIET MEAL
Serve with 3 ounces chunk light tuna in water, drained (120), and 1 cup of grapes (60)

■ **TOTAL MEAL:**

404

CALORIES

Strawberry and Red Onion Salad

Preparation time: 10 minutes / Standing time: 15 minutes / Makes 4 servings

- 3 tablespoons strawberry all-fruit spread
- 2 teaspoons balsamic vinegar
- 1 teaspoon olive oil
- 1 teaspoon organic cold-pressed flaxseed oil
- ⅛ teaspoon salt
- ⅛ teaspoon red pepper flakes
- 1 pound fresh strawberries, hulled and halved
- ¼ cantaloupe, cut into cubes
- ½ small red bell pepper, seeded and diced
- ½ small red onion, thinly sliced
- 1 medium head escarole, torn in pieces

MUFA: 1 cup diced avocado

Freshly ground black pepper

1. In a medium bowl, combine the all-fruit spread, vinegar, olive oil, flaxseed oil, salt, and red pepper flakes until well blended. Gently fold in the strawberries, cantaloupe, bell pepper, and onion. Cover and let stand for 15 minutes to allow the flavors to blend.

2. Place the escarole in a serving bowl. Add the avocado and the strawberry mixture and toss to coat. Season with black pepper to taste and divide evenly among 4 plates.

■ **Eat One Serving:**

186

CALORIES,

4 g protein, 28 g carbohydrates, 8.5 g fat, 1 g saturated fat, 0 mg cholesterol, 111 mg sodium, 9 g fiber

MAKE IT A FLAT BELLY DIET MEAL

Serve with 3 ounces grilled chicken breast (90) and ⅔ cup frozen Cascadian Farm® Edamame, thawed (120)

■ **TOTAL MEAL:**

396

CALORIES

Crisp Romaine Salad with Chicken and Mango

Preparation time: 25 minutes / Cooking time: 15 minutes / Makes 4 servings

2 tablespoons olive oil, divided

3 boneless, skinless chicken breast halves, trimmed (6 ounces each)

½ teaspoon salt, divided

¼ teaspoon freshly ground black pepper, divided

2 shallots, finely chopped

2 tablespoons balsamic vinegar, divided

4 cups shredded romaine lettuce

1 small bunch watercress, large stems discarded

½ cup finely shredded red cabbage

1 firm ripe mango, pitted, peeled and cut into ½" pieces

MUFA: ½ cup pumpkin seeds, toasted

1. Heat 1 tablespoon oil in a large nonstick skillet over medium heat. Season both sides of the chicken with ¼ teaspoon salt and ⅛ teaspoon pepper. Cook, turning once, about 6 minutes on each side, or until a thermometer inserted in the thickest portion registers 160°F. Transfer to a plate; cover and chill completely.

2. Add the shallots and 1 tablespoon vinegar to the skillet and cook, stirring, for about 3 minutes, or until the liquid is almost evaporated. Transfer to a small bowl. Whisk in the remaining 1 tablespoon oil, 1 tablespoon vinegar, ¼ teaspoon salt, and ⅛ teaspoon pepper.

3. In a serving bowl, toss together the romaine, watercress, cabbage, and mango. Cut the chicken diagonally into long, thin strips. Add to the romaine mixture and toss with dressing and pumpkin seeds.

■ **Eat One Serving:**

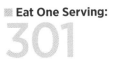

CALORIES,
33 g protein, 19 g carbohydrates, 10.5 g fat, 2 g saturated fat, 74 mg cholesterol, 384 mg sodium, 3 g fiber

MAKE IT A FLAT BELLY DIET MEAL
Serve with 3 Ry Krisp® crackers (105)

■ **TOTAL MEAL:**

406

CALORIES

Greek Lemon Chicken

Preparation time: 18 minutes / Cooking time: 45 minutes / Makes 4 servings

4 skinless, split, bone-in chicken breasts, trimmed (about 1½ pounds)

1 medium red bell pepper, seeded and cut into 8 wedges

1 medium orange bell pepper, seeded and cut into 8 wedges

1 medium Yukon gold potato, cut into 8 wedges

1 medium red onion, peeled and cut into 8 wedges

MUFA: 40 pitted kalamata olives, smashed (about 1⅓ cups)

1 tablespoon extra virgin olive oil
Grated zest and juice of 1 lemon

1 tablespoon minced garlic

1 tablespoon chopped fresh oregano, or 1 teaspoon dried

¾ teaspoon freshly ground black pepper

¾ teaspoon paprika

1. Preheat the oven to 400°F. Tear off 2 sheets of nonstick aluminum foil, each 24" long. Put dull (nonstick) sides together, and fold over the edge on one side twice to make a seam. Open up and line and cover the edges of a 17" by 12" rimmed baking pan (the foil's dull side should face up).

2. Place the chicken on one side of the pan and the bell peppers, potatoes, onion, and olives on the other. In a bowl, whisk together the oil, lemon zest and juice, garlic, oregano, salt, black pepper, and paprika. Drizzle over the chicken and vegetables, and toss to coat.

3. Roast for 40 to 45 minutes, turning the chicken and vegetables halfway through cooking, or until a meat thermometer registers 165°F when inserted into the thickest part of the chicken. Arrange 1 chicken breast and ¼ of the vegetables on 4 plates.

■ Eat One Serving:

401

CALORIES,
39 g protein, 19 g carbohydrates, 18 g fat, 2.5 g saturated fat, 115 mg cholesterol, 742 mg sodium, 3 g fiber

A SINGLE SERVING OF THIS RECIPE COUNTS AS A FLAT BELLY DIET MEAL WITHOUT ANY ADD-ONS!

Spinach-Stuffed Chicken Roulade

Preparation time: 8 minutes / Cooking time: 25 minutes / Makes 4 servings

¼ cup finely chopped onion

1 clove garlic, minced

¼ teaspoon red pepper flakes (or to taste)

2 teaspoons olive oil, divided

1 tablespoon water

¼ cup grated Parmesan cheese

1 package (10 ounces) frozen chopped spinach, thawed, drained, and squeezed dry

4 chicken breast cutlets (about 1 pound)

2 tablespoons minced dry-packed sun-dried tomatoes

½ cup low-sodium chicken broth

MUFA: ½ cup pine nuts, toasted

1. In a medium nonstick skillet over medium heat, cook the onion, garlic, and pepper flakes in 1 teaspoon oil for 30 seconds. Reduce the heat to low, cover, and cook, stirring once, for about 3 minutes, or until softened. In a small bowl, combine the onion mixture, Parmesan, and spinach.

2. Lay the chicken on a work surface, smooth side down. Sprinkle the tomatoes evenly on the chicken. Spread the spinach mixture evenly over cutlets. Roll up the cutlet, ending with narrow tip, and secure with wooden picks.

3. Add the remaining oil to the skillet set over medium heat. Add the chicken and cook about 10 minutes. Add the broth. Cover and cook over low heat for about 7 minutes. Transfer the roulades to a serving platter. Cover to keep warm. Boil the juices in the skillet for about 5 minutes. Cut the roulades into diagonal slices. Drizzle with the pan juices and sprinkle with nuts.

■ **Eat One Serving:**

322

CALORIES,
33 g protein, 8 g carbohydrates, 17 g fat, 2.5 g saturated fat, 70 mg cholesterol, 302 mg sodium, 2 g fiber

MAKE IT A FLAT BELLY DIET MEAL
Serve with 1 medium orange (70)

■ **TOTAL MEAL:**

392

CALORIES

Chicken with Citrus-Avocado Salsa

Preparation time: 8 minutes / Cooking time: 15 minutes / Makes 4 servings

4 boneless, skinless
chicken breast halves
(about 1½ pounds)
4 cups water
½ teaspoon plus
⅛ teaspoon salt
1 ruby red grapefruit

**MUFA: 1 cup diced
avocado**

4 radishes, thinly sliced
¼ cup chopped basil
leaves
Fresh basil (optional)

1. In a large saucepan, combine the chicken, water, and ½ teaspoon salt. Cover and bring to a boil over high heat. Turn off the heat and let sit for 15 minutes, or until a thermometer inserted in the thickest portion registers 165°F.

2. Meanwhile, with a knife, remove the peel and pith from the grapefruit. Working over a bowl to catch the juice, free each segment from its membrane and cut the segments into bite-size pieces, dropping them into the bowl. Add the avocado, radishes, basil, and the remaining ⅛ teaspoon salt. Gently toss to mix.

3. Drain the chicken breasts, discarding the liquid. Cut crosswise into ½" slices. Divide the grapefruit mixture on 4 plates and add one piece of the chicken to each, drizzling the chicken with juice from mixture. Garnish with basil leaves, if using.

■ **Eat One Serving:**

269

CALORIES,
41 g protein, 9 g carbohydrates, 7.5 g fat, 1.5 g saturated fat, 99 mg cholesterol, 188 mg sodium, 3 g fiber

MAKE IT A FLAT BELLY DIET MEAL
Serve with ½ cup steamed brown rice (108)

■ **TOTAL MEAL:**

377

CALORIES

Grilled Ginger-Soy Chicken

Preparation time: 10 minutes / Marinating time: 2 hours
Cooking time: 20 minutes / Makes 8 servings

¼ cup reduced-sodium soy sauce

2 tablespoons minced fresh ginger

2 tablespoons honey

2 tablespoons miso paste

1 tablespoon minced garlic

2 teaspoons toasted sesame oil

¼ teaspoon red pepper flakes

8 boneless, skinless chicken breast halves (3–4 pounds total)

½ teaspoon kosher salt

MUFA: 1 cup unsalted dry-roasted peanuts

1. In a large resealable plastic storage bag, combine the first seven ingredients. Add the chicken and turn to coat. Seal and chill for at least 2 hours.

2. Lightly coat a grill rack with vegetable oil spray. Heat the grill to medium for indirect heat. (If using a charcoal grill, position the coals on one half of grill. If using a gas grill, heat one side to high, the other to low.)

3. Remove the chicken from the marinade. Discard the marinade. Season the chicken with kosher salt.

4. Place the chicken on the hottest section of the grill. Cook for 10 minutes, turning once. Move to the cooler section of the grill and cook 10 minutes, or until a thermometer inserted into the thickest part of the chicken registers 165°F. Sprinkle with peanuts.

■ **Eat One Serving:**

317

CALORIES,
44 g protein, 8 g carbohydrates, 12 g fat, 2 g saturated fat, 99 mg cholesterol, 424 mg sodium, 2 g fiber

MAKE IT A FLAT BELLY DIET MEAL
Serve with 1 cup sliced red peppers (40) with 2 tablespoons hummus for dipping (50)

■ **TOTAL MEAL:**

407

CALORIES

Grilled Oregano Chicken

Preparation time: 10 minutes / Marinating time: 2 hours
Cooking time: 17 minutes / Makes 6 servings

6 small boneless, skinless chicken breast halves (about 2¼ pounds)
1 cup coarsely chopped fresh oregano leaves
4 scallions, trimmed and thinly sliced
½ cup balsamic vinegar

MUFA: ⅓ cup extra virgin olive oil

2 teaspoons freshly ground black pepper
¾ teaspoon salt

1. Place the chicken breast halves between 2 sheets of plastic wrap. Using a mallet or heavy pan, pound to ¾" thickness.

2. In a plastic resealable food storage bag, combine the oregano, scallions, vinegar, oil, pepper, and salt. Add the chicken, seal, and turn to coat. Chill for 2 hours.

3. Lightly coat a grill rack with nonstick cooking spray. Preheat the grill to medium for indirect heat. (If using a gas grill, heat one side to high, the other to low.)

4. Remove the chicken from the marinade, reserving the marinade. Place the chicken on the hottest section of the grill. Cook for 10 minutes, turning once. Move the chicken to the cooler section of the grill and cook for 6 minutes more, turning once, until a thermometer inserted into the thickest part of the breast registers 165°F. Bring reserved marinade to boil for 5 minutes and pour over chicken.

■ **Eat One Serving:**

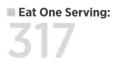

CALORIES,
40 g protein, 5 g carbohydrates, 15 g fat, 2 g saturated fat, 99 mg cholesterol, 410 mg sodium, 0 g fiber

MAKE IT A FLAT BELLY DIET MEAL
Serve with 1 cup grape tomatoes (30) and 1 Laughing Cow® Light Garlic & Herb wedge (35)

■ **TOTAL MEAL:**

382

CALORIES

Lime-Marinated Chicken with Salsa

Preparation time: 20 minutes / Marinating time: 1 hour
Cooking time: 13–15 minutes / Makes 4 servings

4 boneless, skinless chicken breast halves (about 1¼ pounds)
3 tablespoons lime juice (about 3 limes)
2 tablespoons olive oil
1¼ teaspoons ground cumin
¼ teaspoon kosher salt
3 medium tomatoes, chopped

MUFA: 1 cup chopped avocado

½ cup chopped sweet onion (such as Vidalia)
½ cup chopped fresh cilantro
1 small jalapeño chile pepper, seeded and finely chopped

Note: Wear plastic gloves and keep hands away from eyes when handling fresh chile peppers.

1. Put the chicken into a large resealable plastic bag.

2. In a small bowl, whisk the lime juice, oil, cumin, and salt. Transfer 2 tablespoons of the marinade to a medium glass bowl and cover with plastic wrap. Pour the remaining marinade into the chicken bag. Seal and turn to coat. Chill for at least 1 hour.

3. Meanwhile, add the tomatoes, avocado, onion, chopped cilantro, and chile pepper to the bowl with the lime marinade. Toss gently to mix. Cover the salsa and chill.

4. Coat the grill rack or broiler pan with nonstick cooking spray. Preheat the grill to medium-high for direct heat or the broiler to 450°F. Cook the chicken, discarding the marinade, for 6 minutes on each side, or until a thermometer inserted into thickest part of the chicken registers 165°F.

■ **Eat One Serving:**

307
CALORIES,
35 g protein, 10 g carbohydrates, 14.5 g fat, 2 g saturated fat, 82 mg cholesterol, 249 mg sodium, 4 g fiber

MAKE IT A FLAT BELLY DIET MEAL
Serve on a bed of 2 cups baby greens (15) and 2 Ry Krisp® crackers (70)

■ **TOTAL MEAL:**

392
CALORIES

Grape-ful Chicken

Preparation time: 15 minutes / Cooking time: 35 minutes / Makes 4 servings

1 small butternut
squash, peeled,
seeded, and cut into 1"
cubes

1 cup pearl onions,
peeled

4 skinless, bone-in
chicken breast halves
(about 1 pound)

¼ teaspoon salt

¼ teaspoon freshly
ground black pepper

¼ cup chopped fresh
tarragon

2 teaspoons olive oil

1½ cups low-sodium
chicken broth, divided

1 tablespoon cornstarch

2 cups seedless red
grapes

**MUFA: ½ cup walnuts,
toasted and chopped**

1. Place the squash on a microwaveable plate and sprinkle with water to moisten. Microwave on high power for 4 minutes.

2. Season both sides of the chicken with the salt and pepper, and rub with the tarragon.

3. Heat the oil in a large Dutch oven over medium-high heat. Add the chicken and cook for 3 minutes per side or until golden brown. Add the squash, onions, and 1 cup of the broth, and bring to a simmer. Reduce the heat to medium, cover, and cook for 15 minute.

4. Using a slotted spoon, transfer the chicken and vegetables to a serving platter, reserving the liquid in the pot.

5. Dissolve the cornstarch in the remaining ½ cup broth and whisk into the liquid in the pot. Simmer, whisking, for 1 to 2 minutes. Add the grapes. Simmer for 1 minute. Spoon the sauce over the chicken and vegetables. Sprinkle with the walnuts. Serve immediately.

■ **Eat One Serving:**

397

CALORIES,

34 g protein, 38 g
carbohydrates, 14 g
fat, 2 g saturated
fat, 68 mg
cholesterol, 264 mg
sodium, 4 g fiber

**A SINGLE SERVING
OF THIS RECIPE
COUNTS AS A FLAT
BELLY DIET MEAL
WITHOUT ANY
ADD-ONS!**

Almond-Encrusted Chicken Breast

Preparation time: 5 minutes / Cooking time: 10 minutes / Makes 1 serving

5 ounces boneless, skinless chicken breast

1 tablespoon cornstarch

¼ cup fat-free egg substitute

MUFA: 2 tablespoons almonds, finely chopped

1. Sprinkle each side of the chicken breast with cornstarch. Dip the breast into the egg substitute to coat and then sprinkle with almonds.

2. Coat a small nonstick skillet with nonstick cooking spray and heat over medium heat. Cook the chicken for 5 minutes on each side or until a thermometer inserted in the thickest part registers 165°F.

■ **Eat One Serving:**

310

CALORIES,

43 g protein, 10 g carbohydrates, 9.8 g fat, 1.5 g saturated fat, 83 mg cholesterol, 204 mg sodium, 1 g fiber

MAKE IT A FLAT BELLY DIET MEAL

Serve with ¼ cup nonfat cottage cheese (40) and 1 cup grape tomatoes (30)

■ **TOTAL MEAL:**

380

CALORIES

Chicken with Orange Almond Topping

Preparation time: 10 minutes / Makes 2 servings

7 ounces boneless, skinless cooked chicken breasts or cooked chicken pieces, or canned chicken

½ cup mandarin orange segments in light syrup, drained

2 tablespoons orange marmalade

1 tablespoon low-fat red wine vinaigrette
Pinch of ground allspice

MUFA: ¼ cup slivered almonds, toasted

1 tablespoon chopped scallions

1. Cut the chicken breasts into thin diagonal slices. Fan the slices out on 2 salad plates. If using precooked chicken, cut into bite-size pieces. If using canned chicken, crumble into bite-size pieces.

2. In a small bowl, combine the orange segments, marmalade, vinaigrette, and allspice. Stir to mix well and spoon over the chicken. Sprinkle on the almonds and scallions.

■ **Eat One Serving:**

342

CALORIES,
34 g protein, 27 g carbohydrates, 11.5 g fat, 1.5 g saturated fat, 84 mg cholesterol, 169 mg sodium, 2 g fiber

MAKE IT A FLAT BELLY DIET MEAL
Serve on a bed of 2 cups baby greens (15)

■ **TOTAL MEAL:**

357

CALORIES

Chicken with Banana Chutney Topping

Preparation time: 10 minutes / Makes 2 servings

7 ounces boneless, skinless cooked chicken breasts or cooked chicken pieces, or canned chicken

½ medium banana, chopped

2 tablespoons mango chutney

MUFA: ¼ cup cashews, toasted and chopped

½ teaspoon freshly squeezed lemon juice (about ½ lemon)

1. Cut the chicken breasts into thin diagonal slices. Fan the slices out on 2 salad plates. If using precooked chicken, cut into bite-size pieces. If using canned chicken, crumble into bite-size pieces.

2. In a small bowl, combine the banana, chutney, cashews, and lemon juice. Stir gently to mix. Spoon over the chicken.

■ **Eat One Serving:**

337

CALORIES,
34 g protein, 24 g carbohydrates, 11.5 g fat, 2.5 g saturated fat, 84 mg cholesterol, 406 mg sodium, 1 g fiber

MAKE IT A FLAT BELLY DIET MEAL
Serve on a bed of 2 cups baby greens (15)

■ **TOTAL MEAL:**

352

CALORIES

Chicken with Raspberry Topping

Preparation time: 10 minutes / Makes 2 servings

7 ounces boneless, skinless cooked chicken breasts or cooked chicken pieces, or canned chicken

1 cup fresh raspberries

2 tablespoons low-fat raspberry vinaigrette

1/2 teaspoon freshly squeezed lemon juice (about 1/2 lemon)

MUFA: 1/4 cup walnuts, toasted and chopped

1. Cut the chicken breasts into thin diagonal slices. Fan the slices out on 2 salad plates. If using precooked chicken, cut into bite-size pieces. If using canned chicken, crumble into bite-size pieces.

2. In a small bowl, combine the raspberries, vinaigrette, and lemon juice. Spoon over the chicken. Sprinkle with the walnuts.

■ **Eat One Serving:**

305

CALORIES,

34 g protein, 13 g carbohydrates, 14.5 g fat, 2 g saturated fat, 84 mg cholesterol, 154 mg sodium, 5 g fiber

MAKE IT A FLAT BELLY DIET MEAL

Serve with 1/4 cup steamed wild rice (75)

■ **TOTAL MEAL:**

380

CALORIES

Chicken with Honey Mustard and Pecan Topping

Preparation time: 10 minutes / Makes 2 servings

7 ounces boneless, skinless cooked chicken breasts or cooked chicken pieces, or canned chicken

2 tablespoons reduced-fat sour cream

4 teaspoons honey mustard

MUFA: ¼ cup pecans, toasted and chopped

1. Cut the chicken breasts into thin diagonal slices. Fan the slices out on 2 salad plates. If using precooked chicken, cut into bite-size pieces. If using canned chicken, crumble into bite-size pieces.

2. In a small bowl, combine the sour cream and mustard. Stir to mix well. Dollop onto the chicken. Sprinkle with the pecans.

■ **Eat One Serving:**

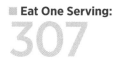

307

CALORIES,

33 g protein, 5 g carbohydrates, 16 g fat, 3 g saturated fat, 90 mg cholesterol, 120 mg sodium, 1 g fiber

MAKE IT A FLAT BELLY DIET MEAL

Serve on a bed of baby greens (15) with 2 Ry Krisp® crackers (70)

■ **TOTAL MEAL:**

392

CALORIES

Zesty Chicken Fiesta

Preparation time: 5 minutes / Cooking time: 10 minutes / Makes 4 servings

2 cups cooked chicken
breast chunks
(10–12 ounces)

1 can (15 ounces)
low-sodium black
beans, rinsed and
drained

1 can (14 ounces) no-
salt-added diced
tomatoes (with juice)

1 tablespoon chili
powder

MUFA: 1 cup chopped avocado

¼ cup fat-free sour
cream

1. In a nonstick skillet, combine the chicken, beans, tomatoes, and chili powder. Bring the mixture to a simmer over medium high heat. Reduce the heat to medium and cook, stirring occasionally, for about 5 minutes. Divide evenly among 4 salad plates and top each with ¼ cup of the avocado and 1 tablespoon of the sour cream.

■ **Eat One Serving:**

298

CALORIES,

30 g protein, 26 g carbohydrates, 8.5 g fat, 1.5 g saturated fat, 61 mg cholesterol, 137 mg sodium, 10 g fiber

MAKE IT A FLAT BELLY DIET MEAL

Serve with 1 cup sliced red bell pepper (40) and 2 tablespoons hummus (50)

■ **TOTAL MEAL:**

388

CALORIES

Tuscan Chicken with Beans

Preparation time: 5 minutes / Makes 2 servings

1 cup cooked, chopped chicken breast (about 6 ounces)

1 cup low-sodium diced tomatoes flavored with garlic and onion, drained

$2/3$ cup no-salt-added canned white beans, rinsed and drained

2 teaspoons balsamic vinegar

1 cup salad greens

MUFA: ¼ cup slivered almonds, toasted

1. In a bowl, toss together the chicken, tomatoes, beans, and vinegar.

2. Divide the greens between 2 salad plates and top each with ½ of the chicken mixture. Serve over greens. Sprinkle with the almonds.

■ **Eat One Serving:**

294

CALORIES,
29 g protein, 25 g carbohydrates, 9.5 g fat, 1 g saturated fat, 54 mg cholesterol, 112 mg sodium, 9 g fiber

MAKE IT A FLAT BELLY DIET MEAL
Serve with ¼ cup steamed wild rice (75)

■ **TOTAL MEAL:**

369

CALORIES

Hearty Sausage with Brussels Sprouts

Preparation time: 9 minutes / Cooking time: 24 minutes / Makes 4 servings

1 pound low-fat Italian turkey sausage (garlic or mild)

2 teaspoons olive oil

MUFA: ½ cup slivered almonds, toasted

6 whole cardamom pods, cracked

¼ teaspoon ground cloves

¼ teaspoon whole cumin seed

⅛ teaspoon ground white pepper

1½ pounds Brussels sprouts, trimmed and quartered

½ cup low-sodium chicken broth

1. Remove the sausage from the casings and discard the casings. Crumble the sausage meat with a fork.

2. Warm the oil in a 12" skillet over high heat. Add the sausage, almonds, cardamom, cloves, cumin, and pepper. Cook, stirring, for about 6 minutes, or until the sausage and almonds become golden in places.

3. Add the Brussels sprouts and broth. Stir to combine. Cover tightly and cook for 15 minutes, or until the sprouts are tender. Uncover and continue cooking for about 3 minutes, or until most of the liquid in the pan has evaporated. Divide evenly among 4 plates.

■ **Eat One Serving:**

341

CALORIES,

33 g protein, 19 g carbohydrates, 17 g fat, 2.9 g saturated fat, 35 mg cholesterol, 54 mg sodium, 8 g fiber

MAKE IT A FLAT BELLY DIET MEAL

Serve on a bed of 2 cups baby greens (15)

■ **TOTAL MEAL:**

356

CALORIES

Steamed Salmon with Snow Peas

Preparation time: 10 minutes / Cooking time: 12 minutes / Makes 4 servings

4 skinless salmon fillets, about 1½" thick (1–1½ pounds)

1 teaspoon grated fresh ginger

1 clove garlic, minced

1 tablespoon freshly squeezed lime juice (about 2 limes)

2 teaspoons reduced-sodium soy sauce

1 teaspoon toasted sesame oil

2 scallions, thinly sliced

1 pound snow peas, trimmed

MUFA: 1 cup chopped avocado

1. Rub the fillets with the ginger and garlic. Coat a steamer basket with nonstick cooking spray and arrange the fillets in the basket.

2. In a saucepan, bring 2" of water to a boil. Place the steamer basket in the saucepan and cover. Cook for 8 minutes.

3. Meanwhile, in a small bowl, whisk together the lime juice, soy sauce, oil, and scallions. Set aside.

4. After the salmon has cooked for 8 minutes, top with the snow peas and cover. Cook for about 4 minutes, until the salmon is opaque and the snow peas are crisp-tender.

5. Make a bed of the snow peas on 4 plates, top with the salmon, sprinkle with the avocado, drizzle with the reserved sauce.

■ **Eat One Serving:**

330

CALORIES,

27 g protein, 13 g carbohydrates, 19 g fat, 3.5 g saturated fat, 67 mg cholesterol, 176 mg sodium, 6 g fiber

MAKE IT A FLAT BELLY DIET MEAL

Serve with 1 medium orange (70)

■ **TOTAL MEAL:**

400

CALORIES

Fish with Summer Squash

Preparation time: 8 minutes / Cooking time: 40 minutes / Makes 4 servings

1 large red onion,
chopped, divided

MUFA: ¼ cup extra virgin olive oil, divided

1 strip lemon zest, cut
into thin slivers

8 ounces zucchini, cut
into ½" chunks

8 ounces yellow squash,
cut into ½" chunks

1 clove garlic, minced

4 striped bass fillets,
about 1" thick
(1–1½ pounds)

1 tablespoon red wine
vinegar

1 tablespoon water

2 tablespoons finely
chopped fresh mint

1. Preheat the oven to
400°F. Set aside
2 tablespoons of the onion
in a small bowl. Place the
remaining onion in a 13" by
9" baking dish. Add 2
tablespoons of the oil and
the lemon zest. Toss and
then spread in even layer.
Roast, stirring occasionally,
for about 15 minutes, or
until the onion is tender.
Remove the baking dish
from the oven. Stir in the
zucchini, squash, and garlic.
Roast for 10 minutes.
Remove from the oven.

2. Increase the oven
temperature to 450°F.
Push the vegetables to one
side of the dish and add
the fish, arranging it
evenly in the pan. Top with
the vegetables. Roast until
the fish flakes easily with a
fork (8 to 10 minutes for
thin fillets; 12 to 15 minutes
for thicker ones).

3. Meanwhile, add the
vinegar, water, mint, and
the remaining 2
tablespoons oil to the
reserved onion. Serve with
the fish.

■ **Eat One Serving:**

272

CALORIES,
22 g protein, 8 g
carbohydrates, 17 g
fat, 2.5 g saturated
fat, 91 mg
cholesterol, 125 mg
sodium, 2 g fiber

**MAKE IT A FLAT
BELLY DIET MEAL**
Serve with ¼ cup
steamed wild rice
(75)

■ **TOTAL MEAL:**

347

CALORIES

Roasted Fish with Artichokes

Preparation time: 10 minutes / Cooking time: 40 to 50 minutes
Makes 4 servings

2 large red onions, cut into ¼" wedges

MUFA: ¼ cup extra virgin olive oil

1 package (10 ounces) frozen artichoke hearts, thawed (about 2 cups)

1 cup small cherry or grape tomatoes

2 tablespoons chopped parsley

1 teaspoon freshly grated orange zest

1 clove garlic, minced

4 skinless flounder fillets (1–1½ pounds total)

1. Preheat the oven to 400°F.

2. In a 13" by 9" baking dish, combine the onions and oil. Toss and then spread in an even layer.

3. Roast for about 35 minutes, or until the onions are very soft. Remove from the oven and stir in the artichokes and tomatoes.

4. In a small bowl, mix the parsley, orange zest, and garlic. Set aside.

5. Increase the oven temperature to 450°F. Push the vegetables to one side of the dish and add the flounder, arranging it evenly in the pan. Spoon the vegetables over the fish and sprinkle with the parsley mixture.

6. Return the baking dish to the oven and roast until the fish flakes easily with a fork (about 5 minutes for thin fillets; 10 to 12 minutes for thicker fillets). Place the fillets on 4 plates.

■ **Eat One Serving:**

302

CALORIES,
24 g protein, 15 g carbohydrates, 16.5 g fat, 2.5 g saturated fat, 54 mg cholesterol, 181 mg sodium, 6 g fiber

MAKE IT A FLAT BELLY DIET MEAL
Serve with ¼ cup steamed brown rice (50)

■ **TOTAL MEAL:**

352

CALORIES

Grilled Salmon Steak

Preparation time: 5 minutes / Marinating time: 30 minutes
Cooking time: 8 minutes / Makes 1 serving

MUFA: 1 tablespoon canola oil

- 1 tablespoon freshly squeezed lemon juice (about ½ lemon)
  Dash ground red pepper
- ½ teaspoon chopped fresh dill
- 4 ounces salmon steak

1. In a resealable plastic bag, whisk the oil, lemon juice, pepper, and dill. Add the salmon and massage the bag to coat evenly. Seal and chill for 30 minutes.

2. Preheat a grill to medium. Remove the salmon from the marinade. Pour the marinade into a microwaveable bowl. Cook the salmon for 4 minutes on each side, or until opaque. Microwave the marinade on high power for about 1 minute, or until boiling. Drizzle over the salmon.

■ **Eat One Serving:**

335

CALORIES,
23 g protein, 1 g carbohydrates, 26.5 g fat, 3.5 g saturated fat, 67 mg cholesterol, 67 mg sodium, 0 g fiber

MAKE IT A FLAT BELLY DIET MEAL
Serve with 2 cups baby greens (15) tossed with 2 tablespoons Newman's Own® Light Balsamic Vinaigrette (45)

■ **TOTAL MEAL:**

395

CALORIES

Lemony Stuffed Sole

Preparation time: 10 minutes / Cooking time: 7 minutes / Makes 4 servings

1 pound sole fillets

¼ teaspoon salt

⅛ teaspoon freshly ground black pepper

1 cup Summer Squash Sauté (page 224)

1 teaspoon extra virgin olive oil

¼ cup dry white wine, or 2 tablespoons freshly squeezed lemon juice mixed with 2 tablespoons vegetable broth

1 tablespoon butter

2 teaspoons freshly squeezed lemon juice (about 1 lemon)

½ teaspoon freshly grated lemon zest

1 teaspoon finely chopped fresh parsley

MUFA: ½ cup pumpkin seeds, toasted

1. Season both sides of the fish with salt and pepper. Place 1 fillet on a flat surface and spread 2 tablespoons of the squash evenly over the top, leaving a ½" margin on both ends. Roll the fillet into a cylinder and secure with wooden pick. Repeat with the remaining sole and squash.

2. Heat the oil in a 12" nonstick skillet over medium heat and add the fish rolls, seam side up. Cook for 2 minutes. Add the wine or lemon juice–broth mixture. Reduce the heat to medium low, cover, and cook 5 minutes longer, or until the fish flakes easily with a fork.

3. Transfer the fish to a plate and tent loosely with aluminum foil. Add the butter, lemon juice, and lemon zest to the skillet. Remove from the heat, swirl until the butter melts, and spoon over the fish. Remove the picks from the fish and place each roll on a plate. Sprinkle with parsley and the pumpkin seeds.

■ **Eat One Serving:**

219

CALORIES,

24 g protein, 8 g carbohydrates, 9 g fat, 3 g saturated fat, 62 mg cholesterol, 334 mg sodium, 1 g fiber

MAKE IT A FLAT BELLY DIET MEAL

Serve with 1 cup skin-on cubed roasted red potatoes (100) dressed with 2 tablespoons reduced-fat sour cream (40)

■ **TOTAL MEAL:**

359

CALORIES

Scallop Ceviche

Preparation time: 15 minutes / Chilling time: 1 hour / Makes 4 servings

½ pound bay scallops
3 tablespoons finely
  chopped red onion
1 medium jalapeño
  chile pepper, seeded
  and finely chopped
  (see Note)
  Juice from 4 limes
½ cup roughly chopped
  fresh cilantro
1 small mango, pitted,
  peeled, and diced

**MUFA: 1 cup sliced
avocado**

1. In a medium glass bowl, mix scallops, onion, pepper, and lime juice. Cover and chill for at least 1 hour. The scallops should be opaque to be edible in ceviche, but that does not mean they are "cooked." Handle any fish going into a ceviche with care.

2. Remove the scallop mixture from refrigerator. Drain the juice and discard. Mix in the cilantro and mango. Divide the ceviche evenly among 4 plates. Fan out the avocado slices on the side.

Note: Wear plastic gloves and keep hands away from eyes when handling fresh chile peppers.

■ **Eat One Serving:**

158

CALORIES,
11 g protein, 18 g carbohydrates, 6 g fat, 1 g saturated fat, 19 mg cholesterol, 121 mg sodium, 4 g fiber

MAKE IT A FLAT BELLY DIET MEAL
Serve with 1 Thomas'® Whole Wheat Pita (140) and 1 apple (80)

■ **TOTAL MEAL:**

378

CALORIES

Chai Scallops with Bok Choy

Preparation time: 8 minutes / Cooking time: 12 minutes / Makes 4 servings

2 bags chai tea

2–4 heads baby bok choy, quartered lengthwise or halved if small (about ¾ pounds)

1 tablespoon finely chopped fresh ginger

1 pound sea scallops, halved horizontally

¼ teaspoon salt

2 teaspoons canola oil

⅓ cup light coconut milk

MUFA: ½ cup cashews, chopped

1 lime, cut into 4 wedges

1. Bring ½ cup of water to a boil. Remove from the heat and steep the tea bags for 3 minutes. Remove and discard the tea bags. Reserve the brewed tea.

2. Sprinkle the bok choy with ginger. Steam over rapidly boiling water in a covered steamer for about 8 minutes, or until bright green and easily pierced with the tip of a knife.

3. Pat the scallops dry and sprinkle with salt. Warm the oil in a large skillet over medium-high heat. Add the scallops in a single layer. (Work in batches if necessary.) Cook for 2 minutes on each side, or until opaque. Remove from the pan and set aside.

4. Add the tea and coconut milk to the skillet. Cook for 1 to 2 minutes, swirling the pan and allowing the sauce to thicken. Divide the sauce evenly among 4 shallow bowls. Top with the bok choy, scallops, and cashews. Serve with the lime wedges.

■ **Eat One Serving:**

250

CALORIES,
23 g protein, 12 g carbohydrates, 12.5 g fat, 3 g saturated fat, 37 mg cholesterol, 392 mg sodium, 1 g fiber

MAKE IT A FLAT BELLY DIET MEAL
Serve with ½ cup steamed wild rice (150)

■ **TOTAL MEAL:**

400

CALORIES

Sweet-and-Sour Shrimp

Preparation time: 5 minutes / Cooking time: 6 minutes / Makes 2 servings

½ teaspoon olive oil

8 ounces frozen stir-fry bell pepper strips

⅓ cup apricot jam

2 teaspoons red wine vinegar

6 ounces (1 cup) cooked, peeled, and deveined shrimp

MUFA: ¼ cup unsalted dry-roasted peanuts, chopped

1. Heat the oil in a nonstick skillet over medium-high heat. Add the peppers and cook, tossing, for about 3 minutes, or until hot. Add the jam and vinegar. Cook for 1 minute, or until bubbling. Add the shrimp and cook for 2 minutes, or until bubbling. Divide evenly between 2 plates and sprinkle with the peanuts.

■ **Eat One Serving:**

357

CALORIES,
23 g protein, 44 g carbohydrates, 11 g fat, 1.5 g saturated fat, 166 mg cholesterol, 223 mg sodium, 3 g fiber

MAKE IT A FLAT BELLY DIET MEAL
Serve on a bed of 2 cups baby greens (15)

■ **TOTAL MEAL:**

372

CALORIES

Sizzled Shrimp with Heirloom Tomatoes

Preparation: time: 20 minutes / Cooking time: 12 minutes / Makes 4 servings

2 teaspoons olive oil, divided

1 pound large shrimp, peeled and deveined

2 tablespoons finely chopped oil-packed sun-dried tomatoes

1 medium red onion, chopped

1 cup fresh corn kernels (about 2 medium ears of corn)

3 medium heirloom tomatoes, chopped (about 3 cups)

4 cloves garlic, minced

½ teaspoon salt

¼ teaspoon freshly ground black pepper

½ cup torn fresh basil leaves

½ cup snipped fresh chives

MUFA: 1 cup sliced avocado

1. Heat 1 teaspoon of the oil in large nonstick skillet over medium-high heat. When hot, add the shrimp and sizzle for 1 minute, or until partially cooked. Transfer to small bowl.

2. Add the remaining 1 teaspoon oil to the skillet along with the sun-dried tomatoes, onion, and corn. Cook for 6 minutes, or until the onion and corn are browned. Stir in the tomatoes and garlic. Cook for 3 minutes. Stir in the shrimp and simmer for 1 to 2 minutes, or until the shrimp are opaque.

3. Season with the salt and pepper. Stir in the basil and chives. Spoon the shrimp mixture into 4 shallow bowls. Garnish with the avocado.

■ **Eat One Serving:**

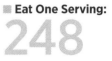

CALORIES,
22 g protein, 21 g carbohydrates, 10 g fat, 1.5 g saturated fat, 168 mg cholesterol, 515 mg sodium, 6 g fiber

MAKE IT A FLAT BELLY DIET MEAL
Serve with 1 Thomas'® Multigrain Pita (140)

■ **TOTAL MEAL:**

388

CALORIES

Sesame Seared Scallops

Preparation time: 5 minutes / Cooking time: 10 minutes / Makes 4 servings

16 sea scallops (about
1 pound)
¼ teaspoon kosher salt
2 tablespoons fat-free
egg substitute
⅓ cup sesame seeds
1 tablespoon peanut oil
1½ pounds baby bok choy
(4–6 heads), quartered
lengthwise

**MUFA: ½ cup sunflower
seeds**

1. Pat the scallops dry and sprinkle both sides with salt. Place the egg substitute in a small bowl. Place the sesame seeds on a small plate. Dip one side of each scallop into the egg substitute and then into sesame seeds. Set aside.

2. Heat the oil in a large skillet over medium heat. Arrange the scallops, sesame side down, with space between them, in the pan. Cook for 3 to 4 minutes, or until the seeds are golden. Flip each scallop carefully without removing the sesame-seed crust. Cook for 6 minutes longer, or until opaque.

3. Meanwhile, put the bok choy into a steamer basket set over a pot of boiling water. Cover and steam for 6 minutes, or until just tender. Nestle the scallops among the bok choy quarters on each of 4 plates. Sprinkle with the sunflower seeds.

■ **Eat One Serving:**

280

CALORIES,
20 g protein, 11 g carbohydrates, 19 g fat, 2.5 g saturated fat, 20 mg cholesterol, 345 mg sodium, 5 g fiber

MAKE IT A FLAT BELLY DIET MEAL
Serve with ¼ cup steamed wild rice (75)

■ **TOTAL MEAL:**

355

CALORIES

Thai Sweet-Hot Shrimp

Preparation time: 15 minutes / Marinating time: 30 minutes
Cooking time: 12 minutes / Makes 6 servings

3 cloves garlic, minced
1 serrano chile pepper, seeded and minced (see Note)
1½ tablespoons reduced-sodium fish sauce (*nam pla*) (see Note)
1½ tablespoons sugar
1 tablespoon freshly squeezed orange juice
1 tablespoon rice wine vinegar
½ teaspoon chile paste
1½ pounds large shrimp, peeled, deveined, and patted dry

MUFA: ¾ cup unsalted dry-roasted peanuts, chopped

1. In a small saucepan over medium heat, bring first seven ingredients to a boil. Reduce heat to medium and simmer for 3 minutes, or until thickened slightly. Remove from the heat and let cool.

2. Place the shrimp in a large bowl. Add 3 tablespoons of the cooled marinade, tossing well to coat. Cover and chill for 30 minutes.

3. Preheat a grill to medium-high. Coat the grill rack with nonstick cooking spray.

4. Thread the shrimp on 6 metal skewers. Grill for 3 to 4 minutes, turning once, until opaque. Divide evenly among 4 plates and sprinkle with the peanuts.

Note: Wear plastic gloves and keep hands away from eyes when handling fresh chile peppers.

Note: Reduced-sodium fish sauce—also called nam pla—*can be found in Asian markets.*

■ **Eat One Serving:**

230
CALORIES,
25 g protein, 9 g carbohydrates, 11 g fat, 1.5 g saturated fat, 151 mg cholesterol, 375 mg sodium, 2 g fiber

MAKE IT A FLAT BELLY DIET MEAL
Serve with ½ cup steamed wild rice (150)

■ **TOTAL MEAL:**

380
CALORIES

Seared Wild Salmon with Mango Salsa

Preparation time: 15 minutes / Marinating time: 1 hour
Cooking time: 15 minutes / Makes 6 servings

SALSA

- 1 ripe mango, pitted, peeled, and diced (about 1½ cups)
- ½ cup chopped red bell pepper, seeded
- ½ cup chopped red onion
- 3 tablespoons freshly squeezed lime juice
- 2 tablespoons chopped fresh mint
- 1 tablespoon finely chopped jalapeño chile pepper (see Note)
- ¼ teaspoon salt

SALMON

- ¼ cup freshly squeezed lemon juice (about 2 lemons)
- ½ teaspoon paprika
- ¼ teaspoon salt
- 2 wild salmon fillets (about 2 pounds, 1" thick)
- 1 tablespoon olive oil

MUFA: 1½ cups mashed avocado

1. To prepare the salsa: In a small bowl, toss together the mango, bell pepper, onion, lime juice, mint, chile pepper, and salt. Cover and chill at least 1 hour to blend flavors.

2. To prepare the salmon: In a large shallow baking dish, combine the lemon juice, paprika, and salt. Place the salmon in the dish and flip to coat both sides. Marinate, covered, for up to 1 hour in refrigerator.

3. Remove the fillets from the marinade. Discard the marinade. Heat the oil in a large nonstick skillet over medium-high heat. Sear the fillets for 15 minutes, turning once, or until opaque. On each of 6 plates, place ⅓ fillet of salmon topped with ½ cup salsa and ¼ cup avocado.

Note: Wear plastic gloves and keep hands away from eyes when handling fresh chile peppers.

■ **Eat One Serving:**

364

CALORIES,

32 g protein, 15 g carbohydrates, 20.5 g fat, 3 g saturated fat, 83 mg cholesterol, 267 mg sodium, 5 g fiber

A SINGLE SERVING OF THIS RECIPE COUNTS AS A FLAT BELLY DIET MEAL WITHOUT ANY ADD-ONS!

Dijon Pork Chops with Cabbage

Preparation time: 18 minutes / Cooking time: 36 minutes / Makes 4 servings

- 4 center-cut boneless pork chops (about 1 pound), trimmed
- 4 teaspoons Dijon mustard
- 1 teaspoon plus 1 tablespoon canola oil
- 1 tablespoon grated fresh ginger
- ½ teaspoon ground cinnamon
- ¼ teaspoon ground cloves
- ½ head red cabbage (about 1 pound), cored and shredded
- 2 Granny Smith apples, peeled and grated
- 1 tablespoon pure maple syrup
- ¼ teaspoon salt
- 2 teaspoons cider vinegar

MUFA: ½ cup pumpkin seeds, toasted

1. Brush both sides of the chops with mustard and set aside. In a large heavy skillet with a lid, warm 1 teaspoon of the oil over medium-low heat. Add the ginger, cinnamon, and cloves. Cook, stirring, for 10 to 15 seconds. Add the cabbage, apples, maple syrup, and salt. Stir, reduce the heat to low, cover, and cook for about 30 minutes.

2. Meanwhile, in a heavy skillet, heat remaining 1 tablespoon oil over medium-high heat. Arrange chops in a single layer. Cook, flipping halfway through, for about 9 minutes, or until a thermometer inserted in the center of a chop registers 155°F.

3. Add the vinegar to the cabbage mixture. Increase the heat to medium. Cook for about 5 minutes, or until most of the liquid evaporates. Place each chop on a plate with a mound of the cabbage mixture. Sprinkle with 2 tablespoons of the pumpkin seeds.

■ **Eat One Serving:**

316

CALORIES,
28 g protein, 25 g carbohydrates, 12.5 g fat, 2.5 g saturated fat, 70 mg cholesterol, 317 mg sodium, 4 g fiber

MAKE IT A FLAT BELLY DIET MEAL
Serve with ¼ cup steamed brown rice (55)

■ **TOTAL MEAL:**

371

CALORIES

Mexican Pork Tenderloin

Preparation time: 10 minutes / Marinating time: 12 hours
Cooking time: 30 minutes / Makes 4 servings

½ medium onion,
chopped

3 cloves garlic, minced

2 chipotle chile peppers
canned in adobo
sauce, finely chopped

3 tablespoons cider
vinegar

2 tablespoons orange
juice

1 tablespoon sugar

2 teaspoons canola oil

1 teaspoon chopped
fresh oregano

1½ pounds pork
tenderloin

½ teaspoon ground
cumin

½ teaspoon salt

¼ teaspoon freshly
ground black pepper

**MUFA: 1 cup sliced
avocado**

1. Coat a small skillet with
cooking spray and cook
the onion and garlic over
medium-high heat for 5–7
minutes. Puree in a blender
with the chile peppers,
vinegar, orange juice, sugar,
oil, and oregano. Place the
pork in a shallow dish and
cover with paste. Cover and
chill overnight.

2. Preheat a grill to
medium-high for indirect
heat. (If using a charcoal
grill, push the coals to one
side. If using a gas grill,
heat one side to high, the
other to medium.)

3. In a small bowl, combine
the cumin, salt, and black
pepper. Remove the pork
from the marinade and blot
dry with a paper towel. Rub
with the cumin mixture. Grill
the pork for 10 minutes.
Move to the cooler section
of the grill. Cover and grill
for 10 minutes more, or
until a thermometer
inserted in the center
reaches 155°F. Let stand for
10 minutes before slicing.
Divide the slices evenly
among 4 plates and top
with the avocado.

■ **Eat One Serving:**

329

CALORIES,
37 g protein, 11 g
carbohydrates, 15 g
fat, 3 g saturated
fat, 111 mg
cholesterol, 416 mg
sodium, 3 g fiber

**MAKE IT A FLAT
BELLY DIET MEAL**
Serve with 1 cup
grape tomatoes
(30)

■ **TOTAL MEAL:**

359

CALORIES

Stir-Fried Rice with Asian Vegetables and Beef

Preparation time 15 minutes / Cooking time 12 minutes / Makes 4 servings

1 pouch (10 ounces) frozen brown rice

1 sirloin or top round steak (8 ounces, 3/4" thick), thinly sliced

2 tablespoons reduced-sodium soy sauce, divided

2 teaspoons canola oil

1 bag (14 ounces) frozen Asian vegetable mix or stir-fry vegetable

1 tablespoon finely chopped fresh ginger

2 teaspoons finely minced garlic

1/2 cup diagonally sliced scallions

MUFA: 1/2 cup dry-roasted unsalted peanuts, coarsely chopped

1. Cook the rice according to the package directions. Set aside.

2. Meanwhile, in a bowl, combine the steak with 1 tablespoon of the soy sauce. Toss to mix. Heat a wok or large skillet over high heat. Add the oil. Place the steak in a single layer and cook without stirring, for 1 minute, to brown. Cook 1 more minute, stirring once or twice, until all the pink in the meat is gone. With a slotted spoon or tongs, transfer the meat to a clean dish and set aside. Add the frozen vegetables to the pan. Cook over medium heat, stirring constantly, for about 5 minutes, or until the vegetables are tender.

3. Add the ginger and garlic to the pan and stir-fry for 30 seconds. Add the steak, scallions, peanuts, rice, and the remaining 1 tablespoon soy sauce. Cook, stirring, for about 2 minutes, or until heated through.

■ **Eat One Serving:**

330

CALORIES,
21 g protein, 30 g carbohydrates, 15 g fat, 2.5 g saturated fat, 27 mg cholesterol, 356 mg sodium, 5 g fiber

MAKE IT A FLAT BELLY DIET MEAL
Serve with 1 medium orange (70)

■ **TOTAL MEAL:**

400

CALORIES

Vietnamese Beef Salad

Preparation time: 15 minutes / Marinating time: 30 minutes
Cooking time: 8–10 minutes / Makes 4 servings

¼ cup reduced-sodium soy sauce

¼ cup freshly squeezed lime juice (about 2 limes)

¼ cup water

2 tablespoons sugar

1 tablespoon minced garlic

2 teaspoons chile paste

½ pound flank steak

6 cups mixed greens

1 cup fresh basil

1 cup fresh cilantro

2 large red onions, thinly sliced (about 1¼ cups)

2 large seedless cucumbers, with peel, julienned

4 medium carrots, julienned

MUFA: ½ cup unsalted dry-roasted peanuts, chopped

1. In a medium bowl, whisk together the first six ingredients. Pour 3 tablespoons into a resealable plastic storage bag. Cover and chill the remaining dressing. Add the steak to the bag, seal, and turn to coat. Chill for 30 minutes.

2. Heat a grill or broiler to medium-high heat. Grill the steak for 8 to 10 minutes, turning once, or until a thermometer inserted sideways in the center registers 145°F for medium rare. Let rest 5 minutes and slice thinly at an angle across the grain.

3. In a large bowl, combine the greens, basil, and cilantro. Evenly divide the greens mixture evenly among 4 plates. Sprinkle on the onions, cucumbers, and carrots. Top each salad with the sliced steak, drizzle with the dressing, and sprinkle with peanuts.

■ **Eat One Serving:**

323

CALORIES,

22 g protein, 30 g carbohydrates, 14.5 g fat, 3 g saturated fat, 21 mg cholesterol, 654 mg sodium, 8 g fiber

MAKE IT A FLAT BELLY DIET MEAL

Serve with 1 cup red grapes (60)

■ **TOTAL MEAL:**

383

CALORIES

Basic Balsamic Flank Steak

Preparation time: 5 minutes / Marinating time: 1 hour
Cooking time: 16 minutes / Makes 4 servings

1 whole flank steak (1½ pounds)
²/₃ cup balsamic vinegar
1 tablespoon freshly ground black pepper
2 cloves garlic

MUFA: ¼ cup olive oil

1. Poke the meat with a fork to help the marinade penetrate. Mix the remaining ingredients in a large resealable bag. Drop the steak into the bag, seal, and refrigerate for 1 hour or up to 24 hours.

2. Preheat a grill to medium for direct heat. Remove the meat from the bag, reserving the marinade. Grill the meat for 6 to 8 minutes per side, or until a thermometer inserted into the thickest part registers 145°F for medium rare. In a small saucepan, boil the reserved marinade for 5 minutes.

3. Slice the meat diagonally across the grain in thin slices and drizzle with the marinade. Divide evenly among 4 plates.

■ **Eat One Serving:**

393

CALORIES,

37 g protein, 7 g carbohydrates, 23 g fat, 5.5 g saturated fat, 56 mg cholesterol, 108 mg sodium, 0 g fiber

A SINGLE SERVING OF THIS RECIPE COUNTS AS A FLAT BELLY DIET MEAL WITHOUT ANY ADD-ONS!

Broccoli and Tofu Stir-Fry with Toasted Almonds

Preparation time: 30 minutes / Cooking time: 12 minutes / Makes 4 servings

4 cups broccoli florets

1 package (1 pound) extra-firm tofu, diced

3 teaspoons toasted sesame oil, divided

1 bunch scallions (about 8), trimmed and thinly sliced

3 cloves garlic, minced

1 small jalapeño chile pepper, seeded and finely chopped (see Note)

3½ teaspoons low-sodium soy sauce

MUFA: ½ cup sliced almonds, lightly toasted

2 cups cooked brown rice

1. Lightly steam the broccoli for about 5 minutes, or until crisp-tender. Set aside.

2. Heat 2 teaspoons of the oil in a wok or large nonstick skillet over high heat. When hot, add the tofu and cook, stirring constantly, for 5 minutes, or until browned. Transfer to a shallow bowl.

3. Add the remaining 1 teaspoon oil to the wok. Heat for 30 seconds. Add the scallions, garlic, chile pepper, and broccoli. Stir-fry over medium-high heat for 2 minutes. Stir in the soy sauce, almonds, and tofu, tossing gently to combine. Divide the stir-fry and brown rice evenly among 4 plates.

Note: Wear plastic gloves and keep hands away from eyes when handling fresh chile peppers.

■ **Eat One Serving:**

360

CALORIES,

21 g protein, 33 g carbohydrates, 18 g fat, 2.5 g saturated fat, 0 mg cholesterol, 184 mg sodium, 7 g fiber

MAKE IT A FLAT BELLY DIET MEAL

Serve with 1 cup sliced red bell pepper (40)

■ **TOTAL MEAL:**

400

CALORIES

Chickpea Salad

Preparation time: 5 minutes / Cooking time: 18 minutes / Makes 4 servings

1 tablespoon olive oil
½ medium onion, chopped
2 cloves garlic, minced
1 teaspoon curry powder
½ medium yellow bell pepper, seeded and chopped
1 can (28–32 ounces) no-salt-added diced tomatoes
1 can chickpeas (16 ounces), rinsed and drained
½ cup fresh or canned chopped pineapple
2 cups thinly sliced fresh spinach

MUFA: 1 cup mashed avocado

1. Heat the oil in a large nonstick skillet or Dutch oven over medium heat. Add the onion, garlic, and curry powder. Cook, stirring occasionally, for about 3 minutes, or until the onion starts to soften.

2. Add the bell pepper, tomatoes, chickpeas, and pineapple. Reduce the heat to medium-low and simmer for 10 to 15 minutes, or until heated through. Stir in the spinach during the last 5 minutes of cooking. Divide evenly among 4 plates and top with ¼ cup of the avocado.

■ **Eat One Serving:**

278

CALORIES,

7 g protein, 35 g carbohydrates, 13 g fat, 2 g saturated fat, 0 mg cholesterol, 319 mg sodium, 10 g fiber

MAKE IT A FLAT BELLY DIET MEAL
Serve with ½ cup cooked Uncle Ben's® Ready Brown Rice (110)

■ **TOTAL MEAL:**

388

CALORIES

Zucchini Rotini

Preparation time: 5 minutes / Cooking time: 10 minutes / Makes 2 servings

¼ cup whole wheat rotini pasta, or any other short shape of pasta

¾ cup 1% fat cottage cheese

1 tablespoon salt-free Italian seasoning

½ cup shredded zucchini

1 cup canned salt-free diced tomatoes, drained

¼ cup reduced-fat shredded mozzarella cheese

MUFA: 20 medium black olives, sliced (about ²/₃ cup)

1. Prepare the rotini according to the package directions. Drain and set aside.

2. In a microwaveable dish, combine the cottage cheese and Italian seasoning. Stir in the rotini and zucchini. Top with tomatoes and sprinkle with mozzarella. Microwave on high for 3 minutes to warm through. Divide the pasta evenly between 2 plates and sprinkle with the olives.

■ **Eat One Serving:**

223

CALORIES,
18 g protein, 20 g carbohydrates, 8 g fat, 2.5 g saturated fat, 12 mg cholesterol, 864 mg sodium, 4 g fiber

MAKE IT A FLAT BELLY DIET MEAL
Serve with 4 ounces sliced Applegate Farms® Organic Roasted Turkey, rolled up (100), and 1 cup sliced red bell pepper (40)

■ **TOTAL MEAL:**

363

CALORIES

Stewed Vegetables

Preparation time: 10 minutes / Cooking time: 20 minutes / Makes 4 servings

MUFA: ¼ cup extra virgin olive oil

1 large onion, chopped
3 cloves garlic, minced
1 can whole tomatoes (16 ounces)
½ teaspoon dried thyme
⅛ teaspoon salt
1 pound green beans, trimmed and cut into 2" pieces
1 medium zucchini, halved and sliced
½ cup chopped fresh basil

1. Heat the oil in a large nonstick skillet over medium heat. Add the onion and garlic and cook, stirring occasionally, for 4 minutes, or until tender.

2. Add the tomatoes (with juice), thyme, and salt, stirring to break up the tomatoes. Bring to a boil over high heat. Add the green beans. Reduce the heat to low, cover, and simmer, stirring occasionally, for 10 minutes, or until the beans are tender.

3. Add the zucchini and cook, stirring occasionally, for 5 minutes, or until the zucchini is tender. Remove from the heat and stir in the basil.

■ **Eat One Serving:**

194
CALORIES,
4 g protein, 18 g carbohydrates, 14 g fat, 2 g saturated fat, 0 mg cholesterol, 242 mg sodium, 7 g fiber

MAKE IT A FLAT BELLY DIET MEAL
Serve with 3 ounces grilled chicken breast (90) and ¼ cup steamed wild rice (75)

■ **TOTAL MEAL:**

359
CALORIES

Stir-Fried Broccoli and Mushrooms with Tofu

Preparation time: 10 minutes / Cooking time: 8 minutes / Makes 4 servings

⅓ cup chicken or
  vegetable broth
1 tablespoon apricot all-
  fruit spread
1 tablespoon reduced-
  sodium soy sauce
1 tablespoon dry sherry
2 teaspoons cornstarch
1 tablespoon canola oil
1 large head broccoli,
  cut into florets
4 cloves garlic, minced
1 tablespoon minced
  fresh ginger
4 ounces fresh
  mushrooms, sliced
1 cup cherry or yellow
  pear tomatoes
8 ounces firm tofu, cubed

**MUFA: ½ cup cashews,
  toasted and chopped**

1. In a cup, whisk together first five ingredients. Set aside.

2. Heat the oil in a large nonstick skillet over medium-high heat. Add the broccoli, garlic, and ginger and cook for 1 minute. Add the mushrooms and cook, stirring frequently, for 3 minutes, or until the broccoli is crisp-tender.

3. Add the tomatoes and tofu, and cook, stirring frequently, for 2 minutes, or until the tomatoes begin to collapse.

4. Stir the cornstarch mixture and add to the skillet. Cook, stirring, for 2 minutes, or until the mixture thickens. Divide evenly among 4 plates and sprinkle with the cashews.

■ **Eat One Serving:**

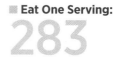

CALORIES,
16 g protein, 25 g carbohydrates,
16 g fat, 2.5 g saturated fat, 0 mg cholesterol,
246 mg sodium,
6 g dietary fiber

MAKE IT A FLAT BELLY DIET MEAL
Serve with 1 medium orange (70)

■ **TOTAL MEAL:**
353
CALORIES

Spaghetti Squash Casserole

Preparation time: 15 minutes / Cooking time: 7 minutes / Baking time: 1 hour
Makes 6 servings

1 spaghetti squash,
   halved and seeded
1 tablespoon olive oil
1 small onion, chopped
2 cloves garlic, chopped
1 tablespoon chopped
   fresh basil, or 1
   teaspoon dried
2 plum tomatoes,
   chopped
1 cup 1% cottage cheese
½ cup shredded low-fat
   mozzarella cheese
¼ cup chopped fresh
   parsley
¼ teaspoon salt
¼ cup (1 ounce) grated
   Parmesan cheese
3 tablespoons seasoned
   dry 100% whole grain
   bread crumbs

**MUFA: ¾ cup walnuts,
   chopped**

1. Preheat the oven to 400°F. Coat a 9" by 13" baking dish and a baking sheet with nonstick cooking spray. Place the squash, cut side down, on the prepared baking sheet. Bake for 30 minutes, or until tender. With a fork, scrape the squash strands into a large bowl.

2. Meanwhile, heat the oil in a medium skillet over medium heat. Add the onion, garlic, and basil, and cook for 4 minutes. Add the tomatoes and cook for 3 minutes.

3. Add the cottage cheese, mozzarella, parsley, salt, and the tomato mixture to the bowl with the squash. Toss to coat. Place in the prepared baking dish. Sprinkle evenly with the Parmesan and bread crumbs.

4. Bake for 30 minutes, or until hot and bubbly. Sprinkle with the walnuts.

■ Eat One Serving:

254
CALORIES,

13 g protein,
20 g carbohydrates,
15 g fat, 3 g
saturated fat,
8 mg cholesterol,
494 mg sodium,
4 g fiber

**MAKE IT A FLAT
BELLY DIET MEAL**
Serve with ⅓ cup
canned Alaskan
wild salmon (120)

■ TOTAL MEAL:

374
CALORIES

Soybeans with Sesame and Scallions

Preparation time: 6 minutes / Cooking time: 14 minutes / Makes 4 servings

1 package (12 ounces) frozen, shelled green soybeans (edamame)
1 tablespoon soy sauce
½ cup water

MUFA: ½ cup slivered almonds

1 dash hot pepper sauce (optional)
2 tablespoons minced scallions
1½ teaspoons toasted sesame oil
⅛ teaspoon freshly ground black pepper

1. In a medium saucepan over high heat, bring the soybeans, soy sauce, and water to a boil, stirring occasionally. Reduce the heat to low and simmer for 12 minutes, or until tender. If any liquid remains, cook, stirring occasionally, over medium-high heat until the liquid has evaporated.

2. Remove from the heat. Stir in the almonds, hot-pepper sauce (if using), scallions, oil and pepper. Divide evenly among 4 plates.

■ **Eat One Serving:**

212

CALORIES,
13 g protein, 12 g carbohydrates, 13.5 g fat, 1.5 g saturated fat, 0 mg cholesterol, 340 mg sodium, 6 g fiber

MAKE IT A FLAT BELLY DIET MEAL
Serve with ½ cup steamed wild rice (150)

■ **TOTAL MEAL:**

362

CALORIES

Balsamic Roasted Carrots

Preparation time: 5 minutes / Cooking time: 25 minutes / Makes 2 servings

8 medium carrots, quartered lengthwise

MUFA: ¼ cup extra virgin olive oil, divided

1 tablespoon balsamic vinegar

½ teaspoon salt

¼ teaspoon freshly ground black pepper

1. Preheat oven to 450°F.

2. In a roasting pan, combine the carrots, 2 tablespoons oil, vinegar, salt, and pepper. Toss to coat. Roast for 20 to 25 minutes, tossing occasionally, until lightly caramelized and tender but still firm. Drizzle with the remaining oil.

■ **Eat One Serving:**

177

CALORIES,
1 g protein, 12 g carbohydrates, 14.5 g fat, 2 g saturated fat, 0 mg cholesterol, 356 mg sodium, 3 g fiber

MAKE IT A FLAT BELLY DIET MEAL
Serve with 2 cups organic mixed baby greens (16), 1 cup halved grape tomatoes (30), and 1 Thomas'® Multigrain Pita (140)

■ **TOTAL MEAL:**

363

CALORIES

Mini Sweet Potato Casseroles

Preparation time: 10 minutes / Cooking time: 10 minutes
Baking time: 10–12 minutes / Makes 6 servings

MUFA: ¾ cup walnuts, finely chopped

2½ tablespoons light butter, melted, divided
1½ pounds sweet potatoes, peeled and cut into ½″ cubes
⅓ cup orange juice
2 tablespoons fat-free half-and-half
½ teaspoon pumpkin pie spice
⅛ teaspoon salt
⅛ teaspoon freshly ground black pepper

1. Preheat the oven to 400°F.

2. Set six 4-ounce ramekins on a sturdy baking sheet. Coat the insides of the ramekins with nonstick cooking spray. In a small bowl, combine the walnuts and 1½ tablespoons butter. Mix with a fork to blend. Divide the mixture among the ramekins and press with a fork to cover the bottoms of the ramekins.

3. Place the sweet potatoes in a medium pot and fill with enough cool water to cover potatoes. Bring to a boil. Cover and cook for about 10 minutes, or until very tender. Drain and place the potatoes in a medium mixing bowl. Add the orange juice, half-and-half, pumpkin pie spice, salt, pepper, and the remaining tablespoon of butter. With an electric hand mixer, beat until smooth. Carefully pour the mixture into the ramekins.

4. Bake for 10 to 12 minutes, or until lightly browned.

■ **Eat One Serving:**

217

CALORIES,
4 g protein, 24 g carbohydrates, 12.5 g fat, 3 g saturated fat, 6 mg cholesterol, 135 mg sodium, 4 g fiber

MAKE IT A FLAT BELLY DIET MEAL
Serve with 4 cups light microwave popcorn (100) and 1 cup sliced red bell pepper (40)

■ **TOTAL MEAL:**

357

CALORIES

Summer Squash Sauté

Preparation time: 10 minutes / Cooking time: 42 minutes / Makes 8 servings

2 tablespoons extra virgin olive oil

6 cloves garlic, sliced

1 teaspoon red pepper flakes

3 pounds assorted summer squash (such as zucchini, yellow crookneck), thinly sliced into disks

½ teaspoon salt

MUFA: 1 cup sunflower seeds

1. In a large nonstick skillet set over medium heat, combine the oil, garlic, and pepper flakes. Cook, stirring occasionally, for 2 to 3 minutes, or until the garlic begins to turn golden. Add the squash and salt. Toss to coat. Cover, reduce the heat to medium-low and cook for 30 minutes, stirring occasionally, until the squash begins to break apart.

2. Uncover the pan and increase the heat to medium. Cook for 10 to 12 minutes longer, or until the liquid is almost gone. Divide evenly among 8 plates and sprinkle with the sunflower seeds.

■ **Eat One Serving:**

156

CALORIES,
5 g protein, 10 g carbohydrates, 12 g fat, 1.4 g saturated fat, 0 mg cholesterol, 156 mg sodium, 4 g fiber

MAKE IT A FLAT BELLY MEAL
Serve with 4 ounces Applegate Farm Organic Roasted Turkey, rolled up (100), 1 cup sliced red bell pepper (40), and ¼ cup hummus (100)

■ **TOTAL MEAL:**

396

CALORIES

Wild Rice, Almond, and Cranberry Dressing

Preparation time: 15 minutes / Standing time: 10 Minutes
Cooking time: 1 hour, 15 minutes / Makes 8 servings

2 cups wild rice

2 strips (½" by 2") orange zest

1 rib celery, 3" of leafy top only

2 teaspoons salt

6 cups water

2 whole cloves

½ small onion, plus 2 cups chopped onions

1 tablespoon olive oil

2 cloves garlic, minced

2 cups seedless green grapes

1 cup unsweetened dried cranberries

1 cup fat-free low-sodium chicken broth

½ cup chopped flat-leaf parsley

MUFA: 1 cup sliced almonds, toasted

1. In a deep, wide 5-quart pot over high heat, bring rice, orange zest, celery, salt, and water to a boil. Stick the cloves into the onion half and add to the pot. Cover and cook over medium-low heat for 35 to 45 minutes, or until the rice is tender. Remove from the heat and let stand, covered, for 10 minutes. Remove and discard the orange peel, onion with cloves, and celery. Set aside.

2. Heat the oil in a large skillet over medium heat and add the chopped onions. Reduce the heat to low, cover, and cook 5 minutes. Increase the heat to medium. Uncover and cook, stirring occasionally, for about 10 minutes. Add the garlic and cook 1 minute. Add the onion mixture, grapes, cranberries, broth, and parsley to the rice and stir to blend. Cover and cook over low heat for 15 minutes. Sprinkle with the almonds.

■ **Eat One Serving:**

322

CALORIES,

9 g protein, 56 g carbohydrates, 8.5 g fat, 1 g saturated fat, 0 mg cholesterol, 655 mg sodium, 6 g fiber

MAKE IT A FLAT BELLY DIET MEAL

Serve with 1 apple (80)

■ **TOTAL MEAL:**

402

CALORIES

Guilt-Free Fries

Preparation time: 5 minutes / Cooking time: 25 minutes / Makes 4 servings

1 large sweet potato and 1 large russet baking potato (1½ pounds total), peeled and sliced into thin strips

MUFA: /₄ cup canola oil

½ teaspoon chili powder
½ teaspoon garlic powder
½ teaspoon ground cumin
½ teaspoon sea salt

1. Preheat the oven to 450°F.

2. In a bowl, toss together the potatoes, oil, chili powder, garlic powder, and cumin. Arrange the potatoes in a single layer on a baking sheet. Bake for 25 minutes. Halfway through, turn the fries over and continue baking.

3. Remove the fries from the oven and place them on several layers of paper towels. Sprinkle with the salt.

■ **Eat One Serving:**

CALORIES,
3 g protein, 28 g carbohydrates, 14 g fat, 1 g saturated fat, 0 mg cholesterol, 338 mg sodium, 3 g fiber

MAKE IT A FLAT BELLY DIET MEAL
Serve with 2 cups mixed baby greens (15) and 1 cup halved grape tomatoes (30) tossed with 2 tablespoons Newman's Own® Light Balsamic Vinaigrette (45) and ¾ cup Cascadian Farm® Organic Sweet Corn, thawed (70)

■ **TOTAL MEAL:**

403

CALORIES

Stir-Fried Asparagus with Ginger, Sesame, and Soy

Preparation time: 5 minutes / Cooking time: 12 minutes / Makes 4 servings

1½ pounds asparagus, trimmed and cut into 2" pieces

MUFA: ¼ cup canola oil

½ large red bell pepper, seeded and cut into strips

1 tablespoon chopped fresh ginger

1 tablespoon reduced-sodium soy sauce

⅛ teaspoon red pepper flakes

2 teaspoons toasted sesame oil

1 teaspoon sesame seeds

1. Bring ¼" water to a boil in a large nonstick skillet over high heat. Add the asparagus and return to a boil. Reduce the heat to low, cover, and simmer for 5 minutes, or until crisp-tender. Drain in a colander and cool briefly under cold running water. Wipe the skillet dry with a paper towel.

2. Heat the canola oil in the same skillet over high heat. Add the bell pepper and cook, stirring constantly, for 3 minutes, or until crisp-tender. Add the asparagus, ginger, soy sauce, and pepper flakes and cook for 2 minutes, or until heated through. Remove from the heat and stir in the sesame oil and the sesame seeds.

■ **Eat One Serving:**

190

CALORIES,
4 g protein, 9 g carbohydrates, 17 g fat, 1.5 g saturated fat, 0 mg cholesterol, 145 mg sodium, 4 g fiber

MAKE IT A FLAT BELLY DIET MEAL
Serve with 4 ounces Applegate Farms® Organic Roasted Turkey, rolled up (100), 1 cup grape tomatoes (30), and 1 medium orange (70)

■ **TOTAL MEAL:**

390

CALORIES

Tuscan White Bean Spread

Preparation time: 10 minutes / Makes 12 servings

1 can (15 ounces) cannellini, navy, or great Northern beans, rinsed and drained
1 large clove garlic
1 tablespoon freshly squeezed lemon juice (about 1 lemon)
2 teaspoons white wine vinegar
2 sprigs fresh flat-leaf Italian parsley
2 basil leaves
1 teaspoon Dijon mustard
¼ teaspoon dried oregano
Red pepper flakes

MUFA: ¾ cup olive oil

Salt
Freshly ground black pepper

1. In a food processor bowl fitted with a metal blade or in a blender, combine the beans, garlic, lemon juice, vinegar, parsley, basil, mustard, oregano, and pepper flakes to taste. Puree until smooth.

2. With the processor or blender running, slowly pour in the oil until it is all absorbed. Season to taste with salt and black pepper.

■ **Eat One Serving:**

140

CALORIES,
1 g protein, 4 g carbohydrates, 13.5 g fat, 2 g saturated fat, 0 mg cholesterol, 87 mg sodium, 1 g fiber

MAKE IT A FLAT BELLY DIET MEAL
Serve with 1 Thomas'® Whole Wheat Pita (140) and 1 cup grape tomatoes (30)

■ **TOTAL MEAL:**

310

CALORIES

Plum and Nectarine Trifle

Preparation time: 35 minutes / Standing time: 30 minutes / Chilling time: 1 hour
Makes 6 servings

3 plums, pitted and
  thinly sliced
2 nectarines, pitted and
  thinly sliced
¼ cup honey
1 tablespoon raspberry
  or white balsamic
  vinegar
1 cup low-fat vanilla
  yogurt
1 cup part-skim ricotta
  cheese
1 fat-free angel food
  cake (10 ounces), cut
  into ½" slices

**MUFA: ¾ cup slivered
  almonds, toasted**

1. In a medium bowl, toss the plums and nectarines with honey and vinegar. Let stand for 30 minutes at room temperature, stirring once or twice.

2. In a small bowl, whisk together the yogurt and ricotta until smooth.

3. Line the bottom of a 2-quart clear glass serving bowl with half of the cake slices. Sprinkle on some of the juice from the fruit. Spread half of the fruit over the cake. Sprinkle on half of the almonds. Spoon on half of the yogurt mixture. Use the remaining cake slices to make a second layer. Top with the remaining fruit. Spoon on the remaining yogurt mixture to cover the fruit. Decorate the top with the remaining almonds.

4. Cover with plastic wrap and chill for 1 hour or up to 24 hours before serving.

■ **Eat One Serving:**
371
CALORIES,
13 g protein, 62 g carbohydrates, 10 g fat, 2.5 g saturated fat, 15 mg cholesterol, 289 mg sodium, 4 g fiber

Chocolate Strawberries

Preparation time: 3 minutes / Cooking time: 8 minutes
Cooling time: 30 minutes / Makes 4 servings

MUFA: 1 cup semisweet chocolate chips

1 tablespoon fat-free milk
20 ripe medium strawberries

1. Line a baking sheet with parchment paper.

2. Place the chocolate and milk in the top of a double boiler set over boiling water. Reduce the heat to medium and allow the chocolate to melt, about 3 minutes. Stir until the mixture is smooth. Remove from the heat.

3. Holding by the stem, dip each berry into chocolate, coating three-quarters of the way up. Place on the parchment, leaving 1" of space around each berry.

4. Chill for 30 minutes to set the chocolate.

■ **Eat One Serving:**

222

CALORIES,
2 g protein, 31 g carbohydrates, 13 g fat, 7.5 g saturated fat, 0 mg cholesterol, 7 mg sodium, 4 g fiber

MAKE IT A FLAT BELLY DIET MEAL
Serve with 1 cup nonfat cottage cheese (160) sprinkled with cinnamon

■ **TOTAL MEAL:**

382

CALORIES

Pumpkin-Maple Cheesecake

Preparation time: 15 minutes / Cooking time: 1 hour and 10 minutes
Chilling time: 4 hours / Makes 12 servings

3 packages (8 ounces each) fat-free cream cheese, at room temperature

$2/3$ cup packed brown sugar

3 large eggs

1 can (15 ounces) pure pumpkin

$1/2$ cup low-fat maple or vanilla yogurt

2 tablespoons all-purpose flour

$1 1/2$ teaspoons ground cinnamon

1 teaspoon ground ginger

1 teaspoon maple or rum flavoring

1 teaspoon vanilla extract

MUFA: $1 1/2$ cups pumpkin seeds, toasted

1. Preheat oven to 350°F. With an electric mixer, beat together the cream cheese and brown sugar until smooth. Beat in the eggs one at a time. Blend in the pumpkin, yogurt, flour, cinnamon, ginger, maple or rum flavoring, and vanilla extract. Pour the filling into a 9" springform pan coated with nonstick cooking spray.

2. Bake 1 hour 10 minutes. Remove from the oven and run a knife around the sides to loosen. Let stand at room temperature for 30 minutes.

3. Chill the cake, uncovered, until cold. Then cover with foil and chill at least 4 hours (or up to 3 days).

4. When ready to serve, carefully remove sides of the pan. Sprinkle each serving with 2 tablespoons of the pumpkin seeds.

■ **Eat One Serving:**

299

CALORIES,
20 g protein, 26 g carbohydrates, 13.5 g fat, 3 g saturated fat, 64 mg cholesterol, 315 mg sodium, 2 g fiber

MAKE IT A FLAT BELLY DIET MEAL
Serve with 1 apple (80)

■ **TOTAL MEAL:**

379

CALORIES

Oatmeal Cookies with Cranberries and Chocolate Chips

Preparation time: 10 minutes / Baking time: 10 minutes / Makes 24 cookies

2 cups rolled oats
½ cup whole grain pastry flour
¾ teaspoon baking soda
½ teaspoon ground cinnamon
¼ teaspoon salt
½ cup brown sugar
⅓ cup canola oil
3 large egg whites
2 teaspoons vanilla extract
¾ cup cranberries, coarsely chopped

MUFA: 2¼ cups chopped walnuts

½ cup semisweet chocolate chips

1. Preheat the oven to 350°F. In a large bowl, combine the oats, flour, baking soda, cinnamon, and salt.

2. In a medium bowl, whisk together the brown sugar, oil, egg whites, and vanilla extract until smooth. Fold in the cranberries, walnuts, and chocolate chips. Gradually fold in the flour mixture and stir until well blended.

3. Drop the batter by tablespoons onto 2 large baking sheets coated with nonstick cooking spray. Bake for 10 minutes, or until the cookies are golden brown.

4. Transfer the cookies to a wire rack to cool completely.

■ **Eat One Serving:**

229

(1 **cookie**):
CALORIES,
4 g protein, 15 g carbohydrates, 11.8 g fat, 1.5 g saturated fat, 0 mg cholesterol, 73 mg sodium, 2 g fiber

MAKE IT A FLAT BELLY DIET MEAL
Serve with ½ cup cottage cheese (80) and 1 medium apple (80)

■ **TOTAL MEAL:**

389

CALORIES

Chocolate Pudding with Bananas and Graham Crackers

Preparation time: 5 minutes / Cooking time: 5 minutes / Chilling time: 2 hours
Makes 6 servings

3 whole graham crackers, crushed
1 ripe banana, sliced
½ cup sugar
¼ cup unsweetened cocoa powder
3 tablespoons cornstarch
Salt
3 cups 2% milk
½ teaspoon vanilla extract

MUFA: 1½ cups semisweet chocolate chips

1. Evenly divide the graham cracker crumbs among 6 custard cups or ramekins. Press the crumbs to cover the bottoms of the ramekins. Top with the banana slices, reserving some for garnish.

2. In a large saucepan, mix the sugar, cocoa, cornstarch, and salt. Stir in the milk. Whisk over medium heat for about 4 minutes, or until the pudding comes to a boil and thickens.

3. Cook for 1 minute longer. Remove from the heat and stir in the vanilla extract. Pour into the prepared custard cups. Chill for at least 2 hours, or until set.

4. Sprinkle each custard with ¼ cup of the chocolate chips and the reserved banana slices.

■ **Eat One Serving:**

398

CALORIES,
7 g protein, 65 g carbohydrates, 15 g fat, 8.5 g saturated fat, 10 mg cholesterol, 147 mg sodium, 4 g fiber

Citrus Ricotta Cannoli

Preparation time: 15 minutes / Makes 12 servings

1 container (16 ounces) fat-free ricotta cheese

1/3 cup confectioners' sugar

1 tablespoon freshly grated orange zest

2 teaspoons freshly grated lemon zest

1 teaspoon freshly grated lime zest

1/2 teaspoon vanilla extract

MUFA: 3 cups semisweet chocolate chips, divided

12 large cannoli shells

1. In a medium bowl, combine the ricotta, confectioners' sugar, orange zest, lemon zest, lime zest, and vanilla extract. With an electric beater, whip until light and fluffy. Gently fold in 2½ cups of the chocolate chips, setting aside the remaining ½ cup.

2. To assemble, spoon the filling into the cannoli shells. Melt the remaining chips and drizzle each cannoli with the melted chocolate.

■ **Eat One Cannoli:**
250
CALORIES,
6 g protein, 34 g carbohydrates, 13 g fat, 7.7 g saturated fat, 6 mg cholesterol, 42 mg sodium, 3 g fiber

MAKE IT A FLAT BELLY DIET MEAL
Serve with 1 cup sliced strawberries (53) and 1 small banana, sliced (90)

■ **TOTAL MEAL:**
393
CALORIES

Double Chocolate Chip Oatmeal

Preparation time: 5 minutes / Cooking time: 5 minutes / Makes 1 serving

Recipe by flatbellydiet.com member Beth Willhite ■ This recipe won our very first flatbellydiet.com recipe contest and was featured online. Said Cynthia, "The combination of freshly ground black pepper and chocolate is absolutely delicious!"

½ cup rolled oats
¾ cup water

MUFA: 2 tablespoons semisweet chocolate chips

¼ teaspoon vanilla extract
⅛ teaspoon freshly ground black pepper
Pinch of salt
2 tablespoons dark chocolate chips

1. In a saucepan over high heat, bring the water to a boil. Add the oats, stir once to moisten, then cook, stirring occasionally, for 3 to 4 minutes, or until the water is absorbed.

2. Remove pan from heat and add the semisweet chips, vanilla extract, pepper, and salt. Stir to thoroughly mix. Spoon into bowl. Sprinkle dark chocolate chips over top while still warm.

■ **Eat One Serving:**

365

CALORIES,
9 g protein, 55 g carbohydrates, 14 g fat, 2 g monounsaturated fat, 6.5 g saturated fat, 0 mg cholesterol, 159 mg sodium, 6 g fiber

MAKE IT A FLAT BELLY DIET MEAL
Sprinkle with ½ cup raspberries, strawberries, or blueberries (30).

■ **TOTAL MEAL:**

395

CALORIES

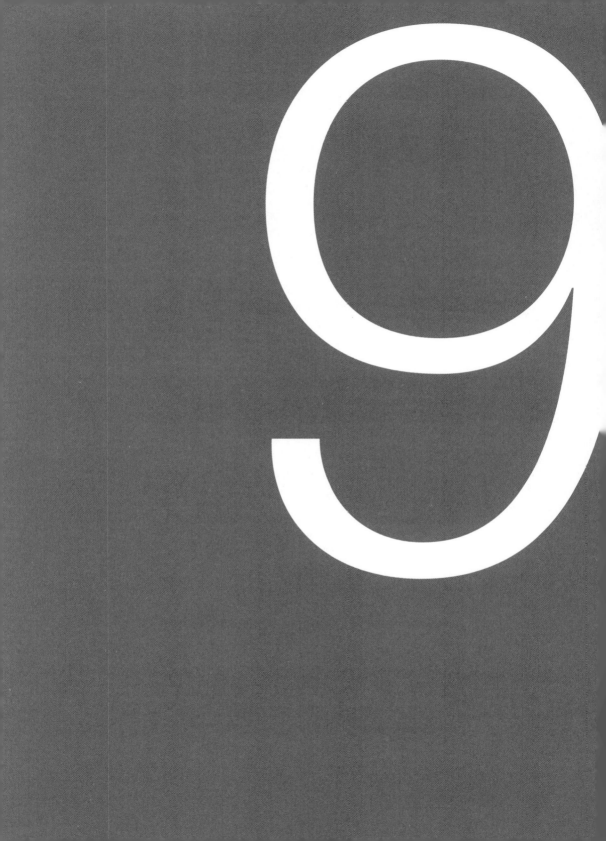

THE FOUR-WEEK
PLAN:
JOURNAL

NOW THAT THE FOUR-DAY Anti-Bloat Jumpstart is under your belt, so to speak, you should already be in the habit of keeping a basic food journal that documents what you eat and how you feel when you're eating it. Recognizing the emotional connection you have with food is critical to losing weight and keeping it off, no matter what plan you're on. But *recognizing* and *fixing* are two different things. During the Jumpstart in Chapter 5, I gave you quick Mind Tricks to help you quickly put the focus back on yourself and your goals every time you came in contact with food. You can use these little strategies anytime, anywhere, to put the breaks on "mindless" and emotional eating. But your relationship to food is a lot more complex than what you do and how you feel when you sit down to a meal. Remember the mirror that sent me careening through a fast-food drive-thru? Sometimes, how you feel about yourself and your body can affect how quickly you succumb to that Big Mac® attack.

Behaviorists now understand how to uncover—and unravel—those mysterious connections. Therapy is one way, if you've got the insurance (or cash) and the spare hour every week to spend trying to remember what you ate 6 days ago and why. Another, more practical way is to maintain a journal. But not just any journal. Most of us have had at least one experience with buying an expensive leather-bound notebook with every intention of capturing our innermost thoughts and feelings, only to find that what we end up with reads like a whole lot of nonsense.

The *Flat Belly Diet* Journal is different. It isn't necessarily a place where you write about the dream you had last night or the fight you keep having with your husband about why he can't seem to do [insert dull but essential household task here.] The *Flat Belly Diet* Journal is the place where you explore your relationship to food, where you attempt to dissect the whys and hows of your eating behavior, and where you try to pinpoint the psychological hot buttons that will help propel you to success. (And success in this context means what? Say it with me: a flatter belly!)

I want you to keep this journal with you and use it every single day of this program. Each day, I will give you an exercise in reflection to help you focus your entry. I call these reflections *Core Confidences* because your confidence level and attitude are at the core of your ability to succeed. There's no need to take all day to complete these exercises. I would never ask you to do anything I wasn't willing—and able—to do, and I certainly can't spend hours a day exploring my relationship to anything. But I can find 15 minutes a day. I can find it on the commuter train or on weekend mornings, just before my girls wake up. If I look for those 15 minutes, I can find them. And so can you.

Core Confidences are essential to forging a true and fruitful mind-belly connection. They will help you discover and understand your motivations, your barriers to success, and the wellsprings of ambition and ability that have driven you to achieve major life goals. It may sound strange, but the same qualities that helped you get that promotion or build a solid relationship with your spouse or raise a healthy, well-adjusted child are what will help you flatten your belly. Confidence, self-awareness, determination, love, acceptance, compassion, organization—if you have any of these qualities, the Core Confidence exercises will help you tap into and exploit them for your belly's benefit.

Make no mistake: Some of the Core Confidences may not be so fun. Some may ask you to confront difficult personal issues or behaviors you might not be proud of. The Core Confidences will help you uncover your demons, confront them, and fight them.

As you fill out these pages, remember to periodically look back and read what you've written in previous entries. That's how you'll spot behavior patterns and notice your progress. Each Core Confidence builds upon the last, moving you closer and closer to a deeper sense of self-awareness. Like life itself, it's hard to know where you're going without knowing where you've been.

As with the journal you kept back in Chapter 5, I have three pieces of advice for you.

- Forget spelling and punctuation.

- Write quickly to ward off your inner critic.

- Speak from your heart.

Now, let's get writing!

DAY 1

■ **CORE CONFIDENCE:** Write down at least three reasons why you have chosen to go on the *Flat Belly Diet*. Describe how you feel about the 28 days ahead and what you expect from yourself.

_____

_____

_____

_____

_____

_____

_____

_____

BREAKFAST

WHAT I ATE:

TIME:	HUNGER BEFORE: -5 -3 0 3 5 7	HUNGER AFTER: -5 -3 0 3 5 7

LUNCH

WHAT I ATE:

TIME:	HUNGER BEFORE: -5 -3 0 3 5 7	HUNGER AFTER: -5 -3 0 3 5 7

SNACK

WHAT I ATE:

TIME:	HUNGER BEFORE: -5 -3 0 3 5 7	HUNGER AFTER: -5 -3 0 3 5 7

DINNER

WHAT I ATE:

TIME:	HUNGER BEFORE: -5 -3 0 3 5 7	HUNGER AFTER: -5 -3 0 3 5 7

■ **CORE CONFIDENCE:** List four things that will help you succeed on the *Flat Belly Diet* (example: "my family's cooperation"). Now write about what you are going to do to ensure that you get each of the four things you need.

_____

_____

_____

_____

_____

_____

_____

BREAKFAST

WHAT I ATE:

| TIME: | HUNGER BEFORE: -5 -3 0 3 5 7 | HUNGER AFTER: -5 -3 0 3 5 7 |

LUNCH

WHAT I ATE:

| TIME: | HUNGER BEFORE: -5 -3 0 3 5 7 | HUNGER AFTER: -5 -3 0 3 5 7 |

SNACK

WHAT I ATE:

| TIME: | HUNGER BEFORE: -5 -3 0 3 5 7 | HUNGER AFTER: -5 -3 0 3 5 7 |

DINNER

WHAT I ATE:

| TIME: | HUNGER BEFORE: -5 -3 0 3 5 7 | HUNGER AFTER: -5 -3 0 3 5 7 |

DAY 3

▓ **CORE CONFIDENCE:** Practice mindful eating. If you watch TV, check your e-mail, even read the newspaper during meals, you will be distracted from how much and how fast you're eating. Have one meal today in total peace and quiet. Take your time; savor the taste and texture of the food and, eventually, the sensation of fullness. Be conscious of the emotions you feel while you eat. Write about the experience.

_____

_____

_____

_____

_____

_____

_____

_____

BREAKFAST

WHAT I ATE:

| TIME: | HUNGER BEFORE: -5 -3 0 3 5 7 | HUNGER AFTER: -5 -3 0 3 5 7 |

LUNCH

WHAT I ATE:

| TIME: | HUNGER BEFORE: -5 -3 0 3 5 7 | HUNGER AFTER: -5 -3 0 3 5 7 |

SNACK

WHAT I ATE:

| TIME: | HUNGER BEFORE: -5 -3 0 3 5 7 | HUNGER AFTER: -5 -3 0 3 5 7 |

DINNER

WHAT I ATE:

| TIME: | HUNGER BEFORE: -5 -3 0 3 5 7 | HUNGER AFTER: -5 -3 0 3 5 7 |

DAY 4

■ **CORE CONFIDENCE:** Think of a meal that didn't go well—maybe you overindulged or ate something you later wished you hadn't. Imagine you could go back and "do over" that meal. Write about what you would do differently next time around.

_____

_____

_____

_____

_____

_____

_____

BREAKFAST		
WHAT I ATE:		
TIME:	HUNGER BEFORE: -5 -3 0 3 5 7	HUNGER AFTER: -5 -3 0 3 5 7

LUNCH		
WHAT I ATE:		
TIME:	HUNGER BEFORE: -5 -3 0 3 5 7	HUNGER AFTER: -5 -3 0 3 5 7

SNACK		
WHAT I ATE:		
TIME:	HUNGER BEFORE: -5 -3 0 3 5 7	HUNGER AFTER: -5 -3 0 3 5 7

DINNER		
WHAT I ATE:		
TIME:	HUNGER BEFORE: -5 -3 0 3 5 7	HUNGER AFTER: -5 -3 0 3 5 7

DAY 5

■ **CORE CONFIDENCE:** Write down two changes you made during the Four-Day Anti-Bloat Jumpstart. How many of these changes turned out to be easier to make than you expected? Describe what happened in each instance.

_____

_____

_____

_____

_____

_____

_____

_____

_____

BREAKFAST

WHAT I ATE:

TIME:	HUNGER BEFORE: -5 -3 0 3 5 7	HUNGER AFTER: -5 -3 0 3 5 7

LUNCH

WHAT I ATE:

TIME:	HUNGER BEFORE: -5 -3 0 3 5 7	HUNGER AFTER: -5 -3 0 3 5 7

SNACK

WHAT I ATE:

TIME:	HUNGER BEFORE: -5 -3 0 3 5 7	HUNGER AFTER: -5 -3 0 3 5 7

DINNER

WHAT I ATE:

TIME:	HUNGER BEFORE: -5 -3 0 3 5 7	HUNGER AFTER: -5 -3 0 3 5 7

■ **CORE CONFIDENCE:** Today, see if you can tell the difference between how it feels to eat when you're feeling hungry and how it feels to eat when you're feeling stressed. Write about those reflections.

_____

_____

_____

_____

_____

_____

_____

_____

BREAKFAST

WHAT I ATE:

| TIME: | HUNGER BEFORE: -5 -3 0 3 5 7 | HUNGER AFTER: -5 -3 0 3 5 7 |

LUNCH

WHAT I ATE:

| TIME: | HUNGER BEFORE: -5 -3 0 3 5 7 | HUNGER AFTER: -5 -3 0 3 5 7 |

SNACK

WHAT I ATE:

| TIME: | HUNGER BEFORE: -5 -3 0 3 5 7 | HUNGER AFTER: -5 -3 0 3 5 7 |

DINNER

WHAT I ATE:

| TIME: | HUNGER BEFORE: -5 -3 0 3 5 7 | HUNGER AFTER: -5 -3 0 3 5 7 |

DAY 7

■ **CORE CONFIDENCE:** Today you cross the finish line for Week One. Well done! List the two or three things you found most difficult about being on the *Flat Belly Diet*. Now write about what you're going to do to clear those hurdles in the week ahead.

_____

_____

_____

_____

_____

_____

_____

_____

BREAKFAST		

WHAT I ATE:

TIME:	HUNGER BEFORE: -5 -3 0 3 5 7	HUNGER AFTER: -5 -3 0 3 5 7

LUNCH		

WHAT I ATE:

TIME:	HUNGER BEFORE: -5 -3 0 3 5 7	HUNGER AFTER: -5 -3 0 3 5 7

SNACK		

WHAT I ATE:

TIME:	HUNGER BEFORE: -5 -3 0 3 5 7	HUNGER AFTER: -5 -3 0 3 5 7

DINNER		

WHAT I ATE:

TIME:	HUNGER BEFORE: -5 -3 0 3 5 7	HUNGER AFTER: -5 -3 0 3 5 7

■ **CORE CONFIDENCE:** Write a personal bio. Who are you? What personal strengths do you bring to your job, family, and health? Then write a bio on the person you aspire to be. Is she more confident, more active, more compassionate? What qualities can you take from the first to help you become the second?

_____

_____

_____

_____

_____

_____

_____

BREAKFAST

WHAT I ATE:

| TIME: | HUNGER BEFORE: -5 -3 0 3 5 7 | HUNGER AFTER: -5 -3 0 3 5 7 |

LUNCH

WHAT I ATE:

| TIME: | HUNGER BEFORE: -5 -3 0 3 5 7 | HUNGER AFTER: -5 -3 0 3 5 7 |

SNACK

WHAT I ATE:

| TIME: | HUNGER BEFORE: -5 -3 0 3 5 7 | HUNGER AFTER: -5 -3 0 3 5 7 |

DINNER

WHAT I ATE:

| TIME: | HUNGER BEFORE: -5 -3 0 3 5 7 | HUNGER AFTER: -5 -3 0 3 5 7 |

■ **CORE CONFIDENCE:** Think back over the last few days. Identify one food-related faux pas (maybe you snuck a few Hershey's kisses from the receptionist's desk at work), and write that on the left side of the page. On the opposite side of the page, jot down everything you can think of that you did right that day (made your child laugh, started a project, took a long walk). Now take another look at the "big picture" of your day. Do you see the one setback in a different light?

BREAKFAST

WHAT I ATE:

| TIME: | HUNGER BEFORE: -5 -3 0 3 5 7 | HUNGER AFTER: -5 -3 0 3 5 7 |

LUNCH

WHAT I ATE:

| TIME: | HUNGER BEFORE: -5 -3 0 3 5 7 | HUNGER AFTER: -5 -3 0 3 5 7 |

SNACK

WHAT I ATE:

| TIME: | HUNGER BEFORE: -5 -3 0 3 5 7 | HUNGER AFTER: -5 -3 0 3 5 7 |

DINNER

WHAT I ATE:

| TIME: | HUNGER BEFORE: -5 -3 0 3 5 7 | HUNGER AFTER: -5 -3 0 3 5 7 |

DAY 10

CORE CONFIDENCE: Today let's focus on what you're grateful for. Keep listing what you love about your body, your family, your job—even your personal surroundings—until your space is filled.

_____

_____

_____

_____

_____

_____

_____

_____

BREAKFAST

WHAT I ATE:

TIME: | HUNGER BEFORE: -5 -3 0 3 5 7 | HUNGER AFTER: -5 -3 0 3 5 7

LUNCH

WHAT I ATE:

TIME: | HUNGER BEFORE: -5 -3 0 3 5 7 | HUNGER AFTER: -5 -3 0 3 5 7

SNACK

WHAT I ATE:

TIME: | HUNGER BEFORE: -5 -3 0 3 5 7 | HUNGER AFTER: -5 -3 0 3 5 7

DINNER

WHAT I ATE:

TIME: | HUNGER BEFORE: -5 -3 0 3 5 7 | HUNGER AFTER: -5 -3 0 3 5 7

DAY 11

■ **CORE CONFIDENCE:** Create a list of five instant indulgences that can be substituted for food when cravings or emotions threaten to get the best of you.

_____

_____

_____

_____

_____

_____

_____

BREAKFAST

WHAT I ATE:

| TIME: | HUNGER BEFORE: -5 -3 0 3 5 7 | HUNGER AFTER: -5 -3 0 3 5 7 |

LUNCH

WHAT I ATE:

| TIME: | HUNGER BEFORE: -5 -3 0 3 5 7 | HUNGER AFTER: -5 -3 0 3 5 7 |

SNACK

WHAT I ATE:

| TIME: | HUNGER BEFORE: -5 -3 0 3 5 7 | HUNGER AFTER: -5 -3 0 3 5 7 |

DINNER

WHAT I ATE:

| TIME: | HUNGER BEFORE: -5 -3 0 3 5 7 | HUNGER AFTER: -5 -3 0 3 5 7 |

■ **CORE CONFIDENCE:** Write a love note to your belly. Include at least two reasons it deserves your affection and respect.

_____

_____

_____

_____

_____

_____

_____

_____

BREAKFAST		
WHAT I ATE:		
TIME:	HUNGER BEFORE: -5 -3 0 3 5 7	HUNGER AFTER: -5 -3 0 3 5 7

LUNCH		
WHAT I ATE:		
TIME:	HUNGER BEFORE: -5 -3 0 3 5 7	HUNGER AFTER: -5 -3 0 3 5 7

SNACK		
WHAT I ATE:		
TIME:	HUNGER BEFORE: -5 -3 0 3 5 7	HUNGER AFTER: -5 -3 0 3 5 7

DINNER		
WHAT I ATE:		
TIME:	HUNGER BEFORE: -5 -3 0 3 5 7	HUNGER AFTER: -5 -3 0 3 5 7

DAY 13

▨ **CORE CONFIDENCE:** To learn more about your food/feelings connection, make four columns, labeled **anger, sadness, fear,** and **happiness**. Remember the last couple of times you craved a food when you were experiencing each of those emotions. Think about what you craved—and ate—and note it in the appropriate column.

_____

_____

_____

_____

_____

_____

_____

BREAKFAST

WHAT I ATE:

TIME:	HUNGER BEFORE: -5 -3 0 3 5 7	HUNGER AFTER: -5 -3 0 3 5 7

LUNCH

WHAT I ATE:

TIME:	HUNGER BEFORE: -5 -3 0 3 5 7	HUNGER AFTER: -5 -3 0 3 5 7

SNACK

WHAT I ATE:

TIME:	HUNGER BEFORE: -5 -3 0 3 5 7	HUNGER AFTER: -5 -3 0 3 5 7

DINNER

WHAT I ATE:

TIME:	HUNGER BEFORE: -5 -3 0 3 5 7	HUNGER AFTER: -5 -3 0 3 5 7

DAY 14

■ **CORE CONFIDENCE:** You've just finished Week Two! Congratulations—you're halfway there! Write about how you feel reaching this milestone. Describe the changes you have noticed this week in yourself and your attitudes toward food and your body—your belly in particular. Outline your expectations for the week ahead.

_____

_____

_____

_____

_____

_____

_____

BREAKFAST

WHAT I ATE:

| TIME: | HUNGER BEFORE: -5 -3 0 3 5 7 | HUNGER AFTER: -5 -3 0 3 5 7 |

LUNCH

WHAT I ATE:

| TIME: | HUNGER BEFORE: -5 -3 0 3 5 7 | HUNGER AFTER: -5 -3 0 3 5 7 |

SNACK

WHAT I ATE:

| TIME: | HUNGER BEFORE: -5 -3 0 3 5 7 | HUNGER AFTER: -5 -3 0 3 5 7 |

DINNER

WHAT I ATE:

| TIME: | HUNGER BEFORE: -5 -3 0 3 5 7 | HUNGER AFTER: -5 -3 0 3 5 7 |

DAY 15

■ **CORE CONFIDENCE:** Identify three or four "high-risk" scenarios—occasions, activities, or places in which you are in danger of eating more than you should or eating the wrong foods. Now create an escape plan that you can implement to avert trouble in each scenario. Write up a description of this plan, using an "If X, then I'll Y" format.

_____

_____

_____

_____

_____

_____

_____

_____

BREAKFAST

WHAT I ATE:

| TIME: | HUNGER BEFORE: -5 -3 0 3 5 7 | HUNGER AFTER: -5 -3 0 3 5 7 |

LUNCH

WHAT I ATE:

| TIME: | HUNGER BEFORE: -5 -3 0 3 5 7 | HUNGER AFTER: -5 -3 0 3 5 7 |

SNACK

WHAT I ATE:

| TIME: | HUNGER BEFORE: -5 -3 0 3 5 7 | HUNGER AFTER: -5 -3 0 3 5 7 |

DINNER

WHAT I ATE:

| TIME: | HUNGER BEFORE: -5 -3 0 3 5 7 | HUNGER AFTER: -5 -3 0 3 5 7 |

■ **CORE CONFIDENCE:** Make a list of at least five activities you've always been interested in but never managed to get around to doing. Rank them in order of preference. Then, alongside each item, enter the very first action you need to take to begin to make it happen.

_____

_____

_____

_____

_____

_____

_____

_____

BREAKFAST

WHAT I ATE:

TIME:	HUNGER BEFORE: -5 -3 0 3 5 7	HUNGER AFTER: -5 -3 0 3 5 7

LUNCH

WHAT I ATE:

TIME:	HUNGER BEFORE: -5 -3 0 3 5 7	HUNGER AFTER: -5 -3 0 3 5 7

SNACK

WHAT I ATE:

TIME:	HUNGER BEFORE: -5 -3 0 3 5 7	HUNGER AFTER: -5 -3 0 3 5 7

DINNER

WHAT I ATE:

TIME:	HUNGER BEFORE: -5 -3 0 3 5 7	HUNGER AFTER: -5 -3 0 3 5 7

DAY 17

CORE CONFIDENCE: Plumb your memory banks for unhealthy eating rules you used to follow (like always cleaning your plate). Where did you learn those rules? How do they continue to affect the way you eat? Now write your "New Rules to Eat By" (for example, "Listen to my stomach and stop eating when it's full").

_____

_____

_____

_____

_____

_____

_____

BREAKFAST

WHAT I ATE:

| TIME: | HUNGER BEFORE: -5 -3 0 3 5 7 | HUNGER AFTER: -5 -3 0 3 5 7 |

LUNCH

WHAT I ATE:

| TIME: | HUNGER BEFORE: -5 -3 0 3 5 7 | HUNGER AFTER: -5 -3 0 3 5 7 |

SNACK

WHAT I ATE:

| TIME: | HUNGER BEFORE: -5 -3 0 3 5 7 | HUNGER AFTER: -5 -3 0 3 5 7 |

DINNER

WHAT I ATE:

| TIME: | HUNGER BEFORE: -5 -3 0 3 5 7 | HUNGER AFTER: -5 -3 0 3 5 7 |

■ **CORE CONFIDENCE:** Make a list of all the things and people you're angry with. Then write next to each, in capital letters: I FORGIVE YOU.

_____

_____

_____

_____

_____

_____

_____

_____

BREAKFAST

WHAT I ATE:

| TIME: | HUNGER BEFORE: -5 -3 0 3 5 7 | HUNGER AFTER: -5 -3 0 3 5 7 |

LUNCH

WHAT I ATE:

| TIME: | HUNGER BEFORE: -5 -3 0 3 5 7 | HUNGER AFTER: -5 -3 0 3 5 7 |

SNACK

WHAT I ATE:

| TIME: | HUNGER BEFORE: -5 -3 0 3 5 7 | HUNGER AFTER: -5 -3 0 3 5 7 |

DINNER

WHAT I ATE:

| TIME: | HUNGER BEFORE: -5 -3 0 3 5 7 | HUNGER AFTER: -5 -3 0 3 5 7 |

DAY 19

▦ **CORE CONFIDENCE:** Try to go through the day appreciating how very much you have. Make a list of five moments you're most grateful for today; read it before you go to sleep.

_____

_____

_____

_____

_____

_____

_____

BREAKFAST

WHAT I ATE:

TIME:	HUNGER BEFORE: -5 -3 0 3 5 7	HUNGER AFTER: -5 -3 0 3 5 7

LUNCH

WHAT I ATE:

TIME:	HUNGER BEFORE: -5 -3 0 3 5 7	HUNGER AFTER: -5 -3 0 3 5 7

SNACK

WHAT I ATE:

TIME:	HUNGER BEFORE: -5 -3 0 3 5 7	HUNGER AFTER: -5 -3 0 3 5 7

DINNER

WHAT I ATE:

TIME:	HUNGER BEFORE: -5 -3 0 3 5 7	HUNGER AFTER: -5 -3 0 3 5 7

▓ **CORE CONFIDENCE:** Give yourself a confidence boost. Make a list of all the new things you're doing that you weren't doing 3 weeks ago. You've probably accomplished a lot more than you think.

_____

_____

_____

_____

_____

_____

_____

BREAKFAST

WHAT I ATE:

TIME:	HUNGER BEFORE: -5 -3 0 3 5 7	HUNGER AFTER: -5 -3 0 3 5 7

LUNCH

WHAT I ATE:

TIME:	HUNGER BEFORE: -5 -3 0 3 5 7	HUNGER AFTER: -5 -3 0 3 5 7

SNACK

WHAT I ATE:

TIME:	HUNGER BEFORE: -5 -3 0 3 5 7	HUNGER AFTER: -5 -3 0 3 5 7

DINNER

WHAT I ATE:

TIME:	HUNGER BEFORE: -5 -3 0 3 5 7	HUNGER AFTER: -5 -3 0 3 5 7

DAY 21

■ **CORE CONFIDENCE:** Welcome to the end of Week Three! Write about how it feels to have come so far. Do you feel empowered? Invincible? Proud? Connected to your belly? Write down all the compliments you've received—including thoughts you've had yourself about how far you've come and how great you look.

_____

_____

_____

_____

_____

_____

_____

_____

BREAKFAST		
WHAT I ATE:		
TIME:	HUNGER BEFORE: -5 -3 0 3 5 7	HUNGER AFTER: -5 -3 0 3 5 7

LUNCH		
WHAT I ATE:		
TIME:	HUNGER BEFORE: -5 -3 0 3 5 7	HUNGER AFTER: -5 -3 0 3 5 7

SNACK		
WHAT I ATE:		
TIME:	HUNGER BEFORE: -5 -3 0 3 5 7	HUNGER AFTER: -5 -3 0 3 5 7

DINNER		
WHAT I ATE:		
TIME:	HUNGER BEFORE: -5 -3 0 3 5 7	HUNGER AFTER: -5 -3 0 3 5 7

▨ **CORE CONFIDENCE:** Write today's entry sitting in front of a mirror. Describe who you see as if you were explaining to a friend what this woman looks like. Be as complimentary as possible.

_____

_____

_____

_____

_____

_____

_____

_____

BREAKFAST		
WHAT I ATE:		
TIME:	HUNGER BEFORE: -5 -3 0 3 5 7	HUNGER AFTER: -5 -3 0 3 5 7

LUNCH		
WHAT I ATE:		
TIME:	HUNGER BEFORE: -5 -3 0 3 5 7	HUNGER AFTER: -5 -3 0 3 5 7

SNACK		
WHAT I ATE:		
TIME:	HUNGER BEFORE: -5 -3 0 3 5 7	HUNGER AFTER: -5 -3 0 3 5 7

DINNER		
WHAT I ATE:		
TIME:	HUNGER BEFORE: -5 -3 0 3 5 7	HUNGER AFTER: -5 -3 0 3 5 7

DAY 23

■ **CORE CONFIDENCE:** If you could have only three foods for the rest of your life, what would they be? Think of a quick recipe—how can you make them fit into the *Flat Belly Diet*?

_____

_____

_____

_____

_____

_____

_____

BREAKFAST

WHAT I ATE:

TIME:	HUNGER BEFORE: -5 -3 0 3 5 7	HUNGER AFTER: -5 -3 0 3 5 7

LUNCH

WHAT I ATE:

TIME:	HUNGER BEFORE: -5 -3 0 3 5 7	HUNGER AFTER: -5 -3 0 3 5 7

SNACK

WHAT I ATE:

TIME:	HUNGER BEFORE: -5 -3 0 3 5 7	HUNGER AFTER: -5 -3 0 3 5 7

DINNER

WHAT I ATE:

TIME:	HUNGER BEFORE: -5 -3 0 3 5 7	HUNGER AFTER: -5 -3 0 3 5 7

CORE CONFIDENCE: In three columns labeled **high, medium,** and **low**, list your motivators in the appropriate column. For example, going down a dress size and being able to walk up a flight of stairs without feeling winded may rank high, while getting a better night's sleep might be a medium.

_____

_____

_____

_____

_____

_____

_____

_____

BREAKFAST

WHAT I ATE:

| TIME: | HUNGER BEFORE: -5 -3 0 3 5 7 | HUNGER AFTER: -5 -3 0 3 5 7 |

LUNCH

WHAT I ATE:

| TIME: | HUNGER BEFORE: -5 -3 0 3 5 7 | HUNGER AFTER: -5 -3 0 3 5 7 |

SNACK

WHAT I ATE:

| TIME: | HUNGER BEFORE: -5 -3 0 3 5 7 | HUNGER AFTER: -5 -3 0 3 5 7 |

DINNER

WHAT I ATE:

| TIME: | HUNGER BEFORE: -5 -3 0 3 5 7 | HUNGER AFTER: -5 -3 0 3 5 7 |

DAY 25

CORE CONFIDENCE: Describe a failure in your recent past. How did you get through it? What was the number one thing that helped you persevere? How can you apply this to your experience on the *Flat Belly Diet*?

_____

_____

_____

_____

_____

_____

_____

_____

BREAKFAST

WHAT I ATE:

TIME:	HUNGER BEFORE: -5 -3 0 3 5 7	HUNGER AFTER: -5 -3 0 3 5 7

LUNCH

WHAT I ATE:

TIME:	HUNGER BEFORE: -5 -3 0 3 5 7	HUNGER AFTER: -5 -3 0 3 5 7

SNACK

WHAT I ATE:

TIME:	HUNGER BEFORE: -5 -3 0 3 5 7	HUNGER AFTER: -5 -3 0 3 5 7

DINNER

WHAT I ATE:

TIME:	HUNGER BEFORE: -5 -3 0 3 5 7	HUNGER AFTER: -5 -3 0 3 5 7

▨ **CORE CONFIDENCE:** Write about a woman you admire. Why is she so special to you? If you could absorb two of her qualities, what would they be and why?

_____

_____

_____

_____

_____

_____

_____

BREAKFAST

WHAT I ATE:

TIME:	HUNGER BEFORE: -5 -3 0 3 5 7	HUNGER AFTER: -5 -3 0 3 5 7

LUNCH

WHAT I ATE:

TIME:	HUNGER BEFORE: -5 -3 0 3 5 7	HUNGER AFTER: -5 -3 0 3 5 7

SNACK

WHAT I ATE:

TIME:	HUNGER BEFORE: -5 -3 0 3 5 7	HUNGER AFTER: -5 -3 0 3 5 7

DINNER

WHAT I ATE:

TIME:	HUNGER BEFORE: -5 -3 0 3 5 7	HUNGER AFTER: -5 -3 0 3 5 7

DAY 27

▨ **CORE CONFIDENCE:** Create a diet motivation booster list: Write down all of the reasons you chose the *Flat Belly Diet*. Be sure to include what you'll get out of changing that's important to you, both **today** and in the **future**. For example: **today**—feel lighter and more energized; **future**—not have to take medication. Reread it periodically as a reminder of something you did for yourself.

_____

_____

_____

_____

_____

_____

_____

_____

BREAKFAST		
WHAT I ATE:		
TIME:	HUNGER BEFORE: -5 -3 0 3 5 7	HUNGER AFTER: -5 -3 0 3 5 7

LUNCH		
WHAT I ATE:		
TIME:	HUNGER BEFORE: -5 -3 0 3 5 7	HUNGER AFTER: -5 -3 0 3 5 7

SNACK		
WHAT I ATE:		
TIME:	HUNGER BEFORE: -5 -3 0 3 5 7	HUNGER AFTER: -5 -3 0 3 5 7

DINNER		
WHAT I ATE:		
TIME:	HUNGER BEFORE: -5 -3 0 3 5 7	HUNGER AFTER: -5 -3 0 3 5 7

■ **CORE CONFIDENCE:** Congratulations!!! You've reached the end of the formal Four-Week Plan. Describe how it feels to have set out to complete this program and to actually reach your goal. How healthy do you feel? How happy are you with your results? Write a pledge to yourself that you will continue to fuel your body and your mind in this healthy way.

_____

_____

_____

_____

_____

_____

_____

BREAKFAST

WHAT I ATE:

TIME: | HUNGER BEFORE: -5 -3 0 3 5 7 | HUNGER AFTER: -5 -3 0 3 5 7

LUNCH

WHAT I ATE:

TIME: | HUNGER BEFORE: -5 -3 0 3 5 7 | HUNGER AFTER: -5 -3 0 3 5 7

SNACK

WHAT I ATE:

TIME: | HUNGER BEFORE: -5 -3 0 3 5 7 | HUNGER AFTER: -5 -3 0 3 5 7

DINNER

WHAT I ATE:

TIME: | HUNGER BEFORE: -5 -3 0 3 5 7 | HUNGER AFTER: -5 -3 0 3 5 7

READ A FLAT BELLY
SUCCESS
STORY

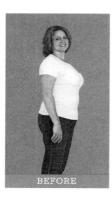

BEFORE

AFTER

Nichole Michl

AGE: 46

POUNDS LOST:

12
IN 32 DAYS

ALL-OVER INCHES LOST:

11

"I LOST 12 POUNDS IN 1 MONTH PLUS 3½ INCHES AROUND THE waist and *many* more inches overall! I was thrilled!" exclaims Nichole Michl.

And well she should be. The 46-year-old graphic designer had tried to lose weight off and on over the years and had even been successful at times. But she could never seem to get rid of her belly fat. "That was always the last to go," she laments. And it was the most annoying to her. So she thought, *"If this* Flat Belly Diet *does what its name says it's going to do—if it's going to help me get rid of my belly fat—I'm going to be one very happy woman."*

Nichole already knew this about herself: When she makes a commitment to something—especially a public commitment—she's more likely to follow it through. So, she challenged herself. "I made the decision to go on the diet—all 32 days' worth—and then I told everyone I knew, so there was no backing out."

She's also the kind of person who, if she commits to something, does it 100 percent. She followed the rules to the letter, she says. "Every single thing they said to do, I did. I bought the right foods. I measured everything. I even followed the diet when I was out, because I know that when you go to a friend's house for dinner, it's so easy to let your guard down—you know, 'I'll try it just this once.' Then, before you know it, you've blown it."

Determined not to let that happen, if Nichole ate at a restaurant, or even if she went away for a weekend, she took along her food in a cooler. "I recently went to a picnic where 50 people sat around eating burgers and other stuff off the grill, and there I was with my little container of food and my bottle of water," she says. "And I looked at what they were eating and what *I* was eating, and I was fine with it. Particularly because so much of what I was eating was organic, and I know that's healthy for me. In fact, I was thrilled with how much of the overall diet is organic."

Nichole calls the support she had during those 32 days a key to her success. Cheered on the whole way by her family and co-workers, she reveled in her weight loss. "You couldn't help but see the changes in my body," she says, "which made me want to keep going. Plus, it was great knowing they were all in my corner."

Being on the diet slowed her down in what she says is a good way. "I had a tendency to eat really quickly—just to get it over with. Like at work. I know you're not supposed to do this, but I always ate at my desk. When I started the diet, though, I learned to pace myself. I thought about what I was eating and truly appreciated every morsel. Even the portions of nuts. Instead of popping a bunch of nuts in my mouth at once, I'd bite off a piece of one, chew it, and really savor it. I try now to do that with everything." She plans to continue with the diet. With this kind of weight loss plus a flatter belly—it's a life plan.

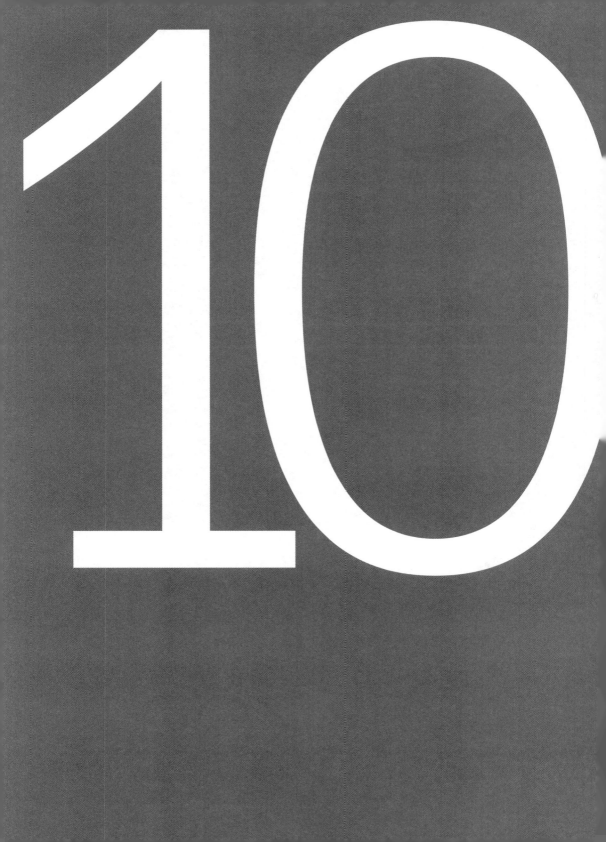

THE FLAT BELLY WORKOUT

THREE YEARS AGO, after nearly 2 months of doctor-mandated bed rest followed by a Caesarean section and the birth of my two daughters, Sophia and Olivia, I was desperate to move again. Prebabies, I had exercised all the time, sometimes devoting 10 to 15 hours a week to working out. I'd run five mornings a week, then walk to work and often take a lunchtime strength-training class at the gym. I religiously attended Thursday night yoga classes for years. (As a friend once said, "When you don't have kids, your day can be as long as you want it to be.")

Then the girls came along, and my whole concept of "me" time changed—forever. Once I was back at work, I had way too much to pack into my 9-hour day to squeeze in a lunchtime workout. Mornings were out: I was up at 5:30 a.m. and racing to catch an early train.

Yoga classes after work? I dashed out every day at 5:15 to get home in time to spend an hour with my girls before they went to bed. Bottom line: I still needed to exercise, but between an hour-a-day commute, children, and a full-time job, it was simply impossible to keep up my pre-pregnancy schedule.

I know from experience how difficult it can be to work exercise into a busy life. That's why it was important to me that the *Flat Belly Diet* include a workout plan that could be tailored to fit any schedule. Even though this diet plan is designed to provide results if you don't exercise, every expert I know firmly believes in the power of aerobic exercise and strength training to boost your mood and energy levels, as well as help you prevent disease and maintain bone and muscle mass as you age. Of course, it will also deliver faster results if you're following the *Flat Belly Diet,* as was demonstrated with our test panelists. Those who added daily exercise lost, on average, 70 percent more body weight and 25 percent more inches than the nonexercisers. While *every single one* of our testers lost fat and inches around their middles—even those who just followed the eating plan—the exercisers lost more and lost it faster.

A Routine Grounded in Science

WHEN I ASKED *Prevention*'s fitness director, Michele Stanten, to devise a companion workout plan for the *Flat Belly Diet,* I knew she'd start by looking for a plan that was backed by the most current research and delivered results. Just like the eating plan, this exercise plan had to be what I call "life-proof." I didn't want any drama attached to it—no running out to buy this or that piece of wacky equipment, no overhauling your basement and turning it into a Pilates studio, no sweating your butt off for months at a time, dreaming of the day you can just lie down in a beach chair and relax already. It had to be a program that most women would find enjoyable and doable within the context of their already busy and demanding schedules. Oh, and I had one more directive for Michele: no crunches.

I don't know anyone who loves crunches. All that straining on your neck and lower back, all that huffing and puffing . . . it just doesn't add up. And truth be told, they're not that effective. In all the research we've seen come out of the exercise labs, the crunch is *never* the move that is found to target ab muscles the best. Over the years, I've met top trainers with the most incredibly defined midsections who tell me they moved on from crunches a decade ago. Today, the truly evolved fitness trainers develop belly-centric workouts that don't focus on just one set of ab muscles but target your whole core—front, sides, and back.

The Flat Belly Workout Basics

THE FLAT BELLY Workout is built around three main components:

- Cardio exercise to burn calories and shed fat
- Strength training with weights to build muscle and boost metabolism
- Core-focused exercises to tone and tighten your midsection

The first part of the plan, **cardio exercise**, burns calories, which is the only way to shrink the layer of fat covering your tummy muscles. Unless you're shedding that fat, you can spend hours doing ab exercises without seeing a change. I rec-

The Exercise Bonus

In a study published in the *Journal of Clinical Endocrinology and Metabolism*,[1] obese postmenopausal women with type 2 diabetes were split into three groups. One group was given a low-calorie diet high in MUFAs that included a nutrition consultation and weekly support meetings. Another group followed a supervised aerobic exercise program consisting of 50-minute walks, three times a week. The third group received both programs. After 14 weeks, the diet-only and exercise-plus-diet groups lost similar amounts of weight, about 10 pounds, but the combo group lost nearly twice as much visceral belly fat.

The Dynamic Duo

If you're going to exercise, I urge you to do both strength training and aerobic exercise. If you're a walker, try the strength exercises in this chapter. If you're all-weights-all-the-time, then add our suggested aerobic routine to your life. The right mix of cardio and strength exercise is important for fast, lasting results. In one study, women in their forties did either straight aerobic exercise (60 minutes, 6 days a week) or a mix of workouts (60 minutes of aerobic exercise, 3 days a week, and 60 minutes of strength training, 3 days a week[2]). After 24 weeks, the combo training group lost 40 percent more weight, three times more subcutaneous fat and—here's the kicker—12 percent more dangerous visceral fat. Even better, they also increased lean body mass such as muscle that fuels your metabolism.

ommend walking for aerobic exercise because it's easy and accessible and offers loads of benefits, but you can do anything you like: cycling, swimming, jogging, or using machines like treadmills, stair climbers, and elliptical trainers.

I'm recommending two types of cardio walks: **Fat Blast** and **Calorie Torch Walks**. Fat Blast walks are steadily paced walks guaranteed to burn off belly fat. The length of these walks will increase each week, and as you become more fit, you should be able to walk at a faster pace (and burn fat faster!) without feeling any extra effort. Calorie Torch walks are set up to be executed in intervals, meaning periodic bursts of fast-paced walking interspersed with a moderate pace. Studies show that interval training keeps metabolism revved up long after the workout is done. The upshot? You burn more calories throughout the day.

If you can't fit in all six cardio workouts every week, don't beat yourself up: Just do what you can. I want you to customize the workouts so they fit your lifestyle. If you're like me, you'll be much more likely to stick with something that you a) *enjoy* and b) *can actually do.* These days, I'm more about walking and hiking (I can bring my girls along) rather than the Spinning classes I attended religiously in my thirties. It's all about what works for you, right now, at this point in your life.

In addition to the daily walk, you'll also be following a strength-training regimen—either **The Metabolism Boost** or **The Belly Routine**.

The Metabolism Boost workout includes four combo moves that target multiple body parts—like your arms and legs—simultaneously. At the same time, they burn more calories overall and in less time (love that). Each of these moves also has a balance challenge, so while you're working your arms, legs, butt, chest, and back, your core will be constantly engaged. Let me repeat that: *Even while you're doing the metabolism-boosting moves, you will be working the muscles of your belly.*

The Belly Routine is nothing less than the best and most effective crunch-free exercise routine ever devised. All of the suggested moves have been lab-tested and shown to be up to 80 percent more effective than traditional crunches.

These workouts are designed to tone and tighten not only your abs but every inch of your body. So wave good-bye to those jiggly trouble spots on your legs, butt, and arms, along with your belly. The beauty of these strength routines is that each has only four or five moves—the most effective ones based on research—so you can get firm fast. You should aim to do three of each weekly. But as I said earlier, if that's not possible, even one or two of each of these routines a week will help to speed up your results. If you do all six workouts one week, make sure to take one rest day each week. It doesn't matter what day you choose; feel free to work it around your schedule.

EXERCISE TIP

If you plan to exercise and have to skip one workout, don't skip **The Metabolism Boost**. In the short term, these are the exercises that will translate into higher calorie burning all day long. Maintaining muscle is essential for preserving lean body mass.

DID YOU KNOW ?

The Importance of Speed and Intensity

IF YOU WANT to lose your belly fat, your "walk" must be aerobic enough to get your heart pumping. That's where speed and intensity factor in. The program we've set out for you incorporates both *steady-paced* and *interval* walks. The steady-paced **Fat Blast** walks are just that. You'll walk at a constant, brisk speed for a certain amount of time, gradually increasing the duration as shown in the plan. And, as you become fitter and your muscles get stronger, you'll naturally walk faster and burn more calories, without it feeling any harder. For instance, a 2-mile walk at 2 mph burns 170 calories (based on a 150-pound person). But when you ratchet it up to 3 mph in that same hour, you'll burn 224 calories—a third more calories, and not an extra minute of exercise time. A win-win situation, don't you agree?

When you do the interval walks—aka **Calorie Torch** walks—you'll be alternating brisk-paced bouts with faster, higher-intensity bursts. In both cases, you can start with the level that is the most comfortable for you and work your way up as you gain more endurance.

Intensity refers to the level at which you perform your exercise. What is high intensity for someone who has not exercised before may be low intensity for someone who works out on a regular basis. No matter what your fitness level, you can get a high-intensity workout simply by pushing yourself just a little out of your comfort zone.

Working at high intensity can burn from 25 to 75 percent more calories than exercising at low intensity. Running, biking, even step aerobics all work the same way. The faster you go or the more effort it takes (say, for example, you're heading up a steep hill), the greater the benefits. You'll be evaluating your level of intensity on a 1-to-10 scale: 1 being how you feel when you're sitting on the couch and 10 being how you'd feel sprinting as fast as you can. It's impossible—and unhealthy—to maintain an extremely high intensity for an entire workout. It's most effective to push yourself into this zone in spurts. Here's how the levels break down:

EXERCISE TIP

Stay Hydrated. Drink at least 2 cups of water about 2 hours before your workout, and then about ½ cup every hour during exercise.

	HOW IT FEELS	INTENSITY LEVEL	SPEED (MPH) *
WARMUP, COOLDOWN	Easy enough that you can sing	3–4	3.0–3.5
BRISK	You can talk freely, but no more singing	5–6	3.5–4.0
FAST	You can talk in brief phrases, but you'd rather not	7–8	4.0+

* Note that these walking speeds are merely guidelines. The fitter you get, the faster you'll walk at each of these levels.

Use these pace and exertion levels (based on a 1-to-10 scale) to ensure that you're working out at the right intensity level for your Fat Blast and Calorie Torch walks.

■ FAT BLAST—Steady-paced walks burn off belly fat. Walk at a brisk speed (5–6 intensity level).

■ CALORIE TORCH—Interval walks raise your calorie burn during and after your workout to shed even more belly fat. Alternate brisk walking (5–6 intensity level) with short bursts of fast walking (7–8 intensity level).

(continued on page 282)

Your One-Month Walking Plan

		WEEK 1	

DAY 1

Fat Blast Walk

TOTAL WORKOUT TIME	HOW IT BREAKS DOWN	INTENSITY LEVEL
30 minutes	3 min warmup 25 min brisk 2 min cooldown	3–4 5–6 3–4

DAY 2

Calorie Torch Walk

TOTAL WORKOUT TIME	HOW IT BREAKS DOWN	INTENSITY LEVEL
25 minutes	3 min warmup 4 min brisk 1 min fast (do brisk/fast intervals 4 times) 2 min cooldown	3–4 5–6 7–8 3–4

DAY 3

Fat Blast Walk

TOTAL WORKOUT TIME	HOW IT BREAKS DOWN	INTENSITY LEVEL
30 minutes	3 min warmup 25 min brisk 2 min cooldown	3–4 5–6 3–4

DAY 4

Calorie Torch Walk

TOTAL WORKOUT TIME	HOW IT BREAKS DOWN	INTENSITY LEVEL
25 minutes	3 min warmup 4 min brisk 1 min fast (do brisk/fast intervals 4 times) 2 min cooldown	3–4 5–6 7–8 3–4

DAY 5

Fat Blast Walk

TOTAL WORKOUT TIME	HOW IT BREAKS DOWN	INTENSITY LEVEL
30 minutes	3 min warmup 25 min brisk 2 min cooldown	3–4 5–6 3–4

DAY 6

Calorie Torch Walk

TOTAL WORKOUT TIME	HOW IT BREAKS DOWN	INTENSITY LEVEL
25 minutes	3 min warmup 4 min brisk 1 min fast (do brisk/fast intervals 4 times) 2 min cooldown	3–4 5–6 7–8 3–4

DAY 7

REST

Fat Blast Walk

	TOTAL WORKOUT TIME	HOW IT BREAKS DOWN	INTENSITY LEVEL
DAY 1	45 minutes	3 min warmup 40 min brisk 2 min cooldown	3–4 5–6 3–4

Calorie Torch Walk

	TOTAL WORKOUT TIME	HOW IT BREAKS DOWN	INTENSITY LEVEL
DAY 2	35 minutes	3 min warmup 4 min brisk 1 min fast (do brisk/fast intervals 6 times) 2 min cooldown	3–4 5–6 7–8 3–4

Fat Blast Walk

	TOTAL WORKOUT TIME	HOW IT BREAKS DOWN	INTENSITY LEVEL
DAY 3	45 minutes	3 min warmup 40 min brisk 2 min cool-down	3–4 5–6 3–4

Calorie Torch Walk

	TOTAL WORKOUT TIME	HOW IT BREAKS DOWN	INTENSITY LEVEL
DAY 4	35 minutes	3 min warmup 4 min brisk 1 min fast (do brisk/fast intervals 6 times) 2 min cooldown	3–4 5–6 7–8 3–4

Fat Blast Walk

	TOTAL WORKOUT TIME	HOW IT BREAKS DOWN	INTENSITY LEVEL
DAY 5	45 minutes	3 min warmup 40 min brisk 2 min cooldown	3–4 5–6 3–4

Calorie Torch Walk

	TOTAL WORKOUT TIME	HOW IT BREAKS DOWN	INTENSITY LEVEL
DAY 6	35 minutes	3 min warmup 4 min brisk 1 min fast (do brisk/fast intervals 6 times) 2 min cooldown	3–4 5–6 7–8 3–4

DAY 7	REST

DAY 1

Fat Blast Walk

TOTAL WORKOUT TIME	HOW IT BREAKS DOWN	INTENSITY LEVEL
60 minutes	3 min warmup 55 min brisk 2 min cooldown	3–4 5–6 3–4

DAY 2

Calorie Torch Walk

TOTAL WORKOUT TIME	HOW IT BREAKS DOWN	INTENSITY LEVEL
45 minutes	3 min warmup 4 min brisk 1 min fast (do brisk/fast intervals 8 times) 2 min cooldown	3–4 5–6 7–8 3–4

DAY 3

Fat Blast Walk

TOTAL WORKOUT TIME	HOW IT BREAKS DOWN	INTENSITY LEVEL
60 minutes	3 min warmup 55 min brisk 2 min cooldown	3–4 5–6 3–4

DAY 4

Calorie Torch Walk

TOTAL WORKOUT TIME	HOW IT BREAKS DOWN	INTENSITY LEVEL
45 minutes	3 min warmup 4 min brisk 1 min fast (do brisk/fast intervals 8 times) 2 min cooldown	3–4 5–6 7–8 3–4

DAY 5

Fat Blast Walk

TOTAL WORKOUT TIME	HOW IT BREAKS DOWN	INTENSITY LEVEL
60 minutes	3 min warmup 55 min brisk 2 min cool-down	3–4 5–6 3–4

DAY 6

Calorie Torch Walk

TOTAL WORKOUT TIME	HOW IT BREAKS DOWN	INTENSITY LEVEL
45 minutes	3 min warmup 4 min brisk 1 min fast (do brisk/fast intervals 8 times) 2 min cooldown	3–4 5–6 7–8 3–4

DAY 7

REST

DAY 1

Fat Blast Walk

TOTAL WORKOUT TIME	HOW IT BREAKS DOWN	INTENSITY LEVEL
60 minutes	3 min warmup 55 min brisk 2 min cooldown	3–4 5–6 3–4

DAY 2

Calorie Torch Walk

TOTAL WORKOUT TIME	HOW IT BREAKS DOWN	INTENSITY LEVEL
45 minutes	3 min warmup 4 min brisk 1 min fast (do brisk/fast intervals 8 times) 2 min cooldown	3–4 5–6 7–8 3–4

DAY 3

Fat Blast walk

TOTAL WORKOUT TIME	HOW IT BREAKS DOWN	INTENSITY LEVEL
60 minutes	3 min warmup 55 min brisk 2 min cooldown	3–4 5–6 3–4

DAY 4

Calorie Torch Walk

TOTAL WORKOUT TIME	HOW IT BREAKS DOWN	INTENSITY LEVEL
45 minutes	3 min warmup 4 min brisk 1 min fast (do brisk/fast intervals 8 times) 2 min cooldown	3–4 5–6 7–8 3–4

DAY 5

Fat Blast Walk

TOTAL WORKOUT TIME	HOW IT BREAKS DOWN	INTENSITY LEVEL
60 minutes	3 min warmup 55 min brisk 2 min cooldown	3–4 5–6 3–4

DAY 6

Calorie Torch Walk

TOTAL WORKOUT TIME	HOW IT BREAKS DOWN	INTENSITY LEVEL
45 minutes	3 min warmup 4 min brisk 1 min fast (do brisk/fast intervals 8 times) 2 min cooldown	3–4 5–6 7–8 3–4

DAY 7

REST

Get Your Walking Form Up to Speed

THE SECRET TO turning your everyday stroll into a fat-blasting stride is proper walking form and technique. The most common mistake people make when they try to pick up the pace is that they take longer strides. This can actually slow you down because your outstretched leg acts like a brake, and it can cause injuries due to increased stress on your joints. Instead, take shorter, quicker steps, rolling from heel to toes and pushing off with your toes. Next, bend your arms at about 90-degree angles and swing them forward (no higher than chest height) and back so your hand is almost skimming your hip. Letting your arms flail across your body will slow down your forward momentum. Practice these techniques and you'll be cruising past other walkers in no time.

Gear Up for Your Walks

YOUR SHOES

Find a knowledgeable salesperson. Unlike mass-market retailers, specialty stores often employ trained shoe fitters who will ask you about your walking habits and watch you walk. This information will improve your chances of getting the right shoe for your feet.

Get your feet measured. Your size can change over time, and footwear that's too small can set you up for an array of problems. Make sure you have a thumb's width of room in front of the end of your big toe while you're standing rather than sitting.

Replace your shoes every 300 to 500 miles. That's about every 5 to 8 months if you're walking about 3 miles 5 days a week. By the time a sneaker looks trashed on the outside, the inside support and cushioning are long gone. I know, it's tough to part with a comfortable pair of old sneakers, but you'll be doing yourself and your feet a favor. Worn-out shoes are a common cause of foot, knee, and even back pain.

YOUR SOCKS

Look for synthetic fabrics that wick moisture away, keeping your feet dry and making them less prone to blisters. Avoid all-cotton socks. Since some are thick and others are thin, wear your walking socks when you try shoes on because they can affect the fit.

The Metabolism Boost: Muscle in on Belly Fat

I'VE ALWAYS BEEN devoted to strength training. (My daughters know that when I leave for the gym, "Mommy's going to make muscles.") It gives me confidence and a sense of empowerment. Plus, I just like the way it makes my body feel: toned, strong, and healthy. I also know how important it is as I get older. Strength training preserves and even rebuilds precious muscle—the body's calorie-burning engine that fuels metabolism. Beginning as early as in your thirties, you start to lose about ½ pound of muscle a year. If you don't take action, that loss can double by the time you hit menopause. With every pound of muscle lost, your body burns fewer calories, which explains why gaining weight gets easier and losing it gets tougher as you get older. Decreasing muscle mass also makes you weaker, and everyday tasks such as getting out of a chair and climbing the stairs become more difficult. As a result, you start to move less—further contributing to muscle loss and fat gain.

When you challenge a muscle, you create microscopic tears in the muscle tissue. (I know the word *tear* doesn't sound all that healthy, but trust me, in this case it is.) Your body then comes to the rescue and fills those crevices with protein, creating new muscle tissue. This is why you should wait a day between strength-training workouts—to give the muscles time to repair themselves.

Replacing the tissue creates stronger muscles—the result you want, because stronger muscle mass makes our bodies look firmer, tighter, and more toned. Most importantly, though, because muscle mass burns about seven times more calories than fat (about 15 more a day per pound), the more muscle you have, the faster you'll burn calories and lose belly fat.

Strength training increases your energy as well, which makes almost every task easier, so you're more likely to remain active throughout the day.

Finally, strong muscles also protect and build strong bones, which is essential, particularly for a woman. As if losing muscle mass weren't bad enough, women start to lose bone in their midthirties as well, a loss that accelerates as they age and gathers even more speed going into menopause. At that point, some women begin to lose up to 20 percent of their bone within the first 5 years. Bone loss can lead to accidental breaks and spontaneous fractures (when bones break for no apparent reason), both of which become harder to heal as we get older, as there is less bone to knit the fracture together. Bone loss also leads to spinal curvature, which, in addition to being uncomfortable, makes standing straight impossible and ultimately causes the belly to protrude. Strength training stresses your bones by stretching and pulling muscles and tendons to increase bone density and reduce the risk of osteoporosis. If you already have osteoporosis, strength training can lessen its impact—but check with your doctor before starting any exercise program.

Here are six other ways strength training can improve your health.

▨ You'll sleep better. People who strength train regularly are less likely to struggle with insomnia.

▨ You'll increase muscle. Each pound burns an extra 15 calories per day.

Ensure Your Safety Outside

- Walk with a buddy.
- Choose routes you're familiar with.
- Wear reflective clothing and carry a flashlight in the dark and at dawn and dusk. Wear bright colors during the day.
- Try to avoid rush hour to reduce your exposure to carbon monoxide.
- Don't carry valuables with you.
- Walk facing traffic so you can see cars coming.
- Carry a cell phone and an ID.
- If you listen to music, keep the volume low enough so you can hear if a car or person is approaching you.

- You'll improve your balance by strengthening ligaments and tendons.

- You'll have more stamina. As you grow stronger, you won't fatigue as easily.

- You'll reduce your diabetes risk. Lean muscle tissue helps your body metabolize blood sugar.

- You'll minimize the appearance of cellulite. Building firm, compact muscle will smooth out lumpy lower-body fat.

Before You Start: Strength-Training Basics

IF YOU'RE NOT yet doing any strength training, *now is the time to start!* If you're currently lifting weights, then try ramping it up a notch.

THE TERMS: If you're picking up dumbbells for the first time, here are some strength- training basics. The word *rep* is short for *repetition*: for example, each time you lift and lower a dumbbell, or roll your upper body off the floor and then lower it back down, it's considered one repetition. A specific number of reps (8, 10, 12, or so) is called a *set*.

YOUR WEIGHTS: Many women train with weights too light to produce the metabolic boost and body firming they want. Don't be afraid of heavier weights—you won't get big, bulky muscles (women simply don't have enough of the hormones needed for those types of results), but you will get stronger and firmer faster. For the best results, the weight you choose should be heavy enough that by your last rep, you feel like you can't do any more using good form. If you can, you need to increase the amount of weight you're lifting. If you can't do at least eight reps, then the weight is too heavy: Choose a lighter weight or try the easier version of the exercise. Because some muscles are bigger than others, you'll need to use heavier weights for exercises that target your chest, back, legs, and butt. For smaller muscles like your arms and shoulders, you'll probably want lighter weights.

■ YOUR ROUTINE: In The Metabolism Boost, you'll begin with one set of 10 reps and progress to two sets of 15 reps during the 4-week program. Remember, if at any point the weight you're lifting isn't fatiguing the targeted muscles by your last rep, it's time to increase the amount of weight you're using or try the harder variation. (For the ab exercises, you can try the harder version or increase your number of reps.)

■ YOUR EQUIPMENT: You will need two sets of dumbbells for this section of the program—light and heavy. If you are a beginner, try starting with a 3-pound and a 5-pound set. If you're more experienced, a 5-pound and 8-pound set is a good place to begin. Remember, these are general guidelines, so adjust the amount of weight you're lifting, based on my recommendations above. It's easy to determine your correct weight: If the set is so easy that you feel at the end that you can keep going, you're probably not working hard enough—that is, you're not doing enough reps or the weights are too light. If, on the other hand, you can barely get the last rep in for the last set, then your choice of weight and pounds is just right. Eventually, as your muscles get stronger, you'll become accustomed to the number of sets and reps you're doing. That's the time to move on.

What time should I exercise?

A: Some surveys have shown that morning exercisers are more consistent because there are fewer opportunities to get sidetracked and skip it than with an evening workout. But if you're not a morning person, the snooze button may be all you need to distract you. The most important consideration should be finding a time when you're most willing and able to exercise. Fit your workouts into your life when it's most convenient for you—otherwise, other activities will always bump exercise off your schedule. There's no significant impact on the calories you burn or how quickly you'll see results based on the time of day you exercise. What matters most is that you *just do it.*

In **The Belly Routine**, we give you a specific number of reps to follow, but you can select from our suggestions for how to make it easier or harder, depending on what works best for you. Just remember that if you want to develop lean muscle tissue, you must select a weight that's challenging.

THE METABOLISM BOOST WEEKLY PLAN

WEEK	DAY 2	DAY 4	DAY 6
1	10 reps	10 reps	10 reps
2	15 reps	15 reps	15 reps
3	2 sets, 10 reps	2 sets, 10 reps	2 sets, 10 reps
4	2 sets, 15 reps	2 sets, 15 reps	2 sets, 15 reps

Lunge Press

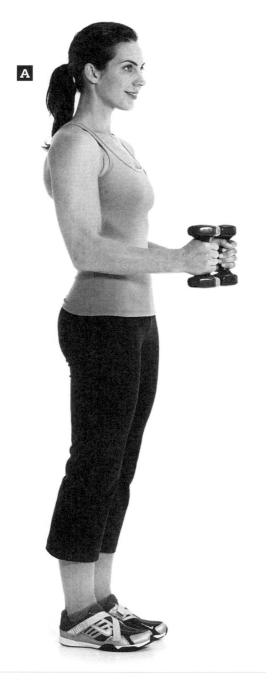

**MAIN
MOVE**

A. Stand with feet together. Holding a dumbbell in each hand, bend arms to 90 degrees so dumbbells are in front of you, forearms parallel to floor, palms facing each other.

B. Step right foot 2 to 3 feet behind you, landing on ball of foot. Bend knees, lowering right knee toward floor until left thigh is parallel to floor. Keep left knee directly over ankle. At the same time, press dumbbells behind you, straightening arms. Hold for a second, then press into left foot, standing back up, bringing feet together, and bending arms back to start position. Do one set, then repeat with opposite leg.

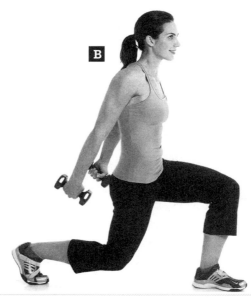

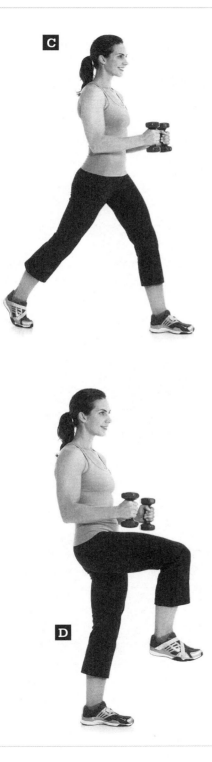

**MAKE IT
EASIER**

C. Do stationary lunges by starting with left foot 2 to 3 feet in front of right foot, right heel off floor. Maintain this position for one set, then switch legs and repeat.

**MAKE IT
HARDER**

D. As you stand back up from the lunge position, raise right knee in front of you to hip height, leg bent 90 degrees. At the same time, bend arms back to start position. Hold for 1 second, balancing on left foot, then swing right foot behind you and repeat. Complete one set, and then repeat with opposite leg.

Squat Curl

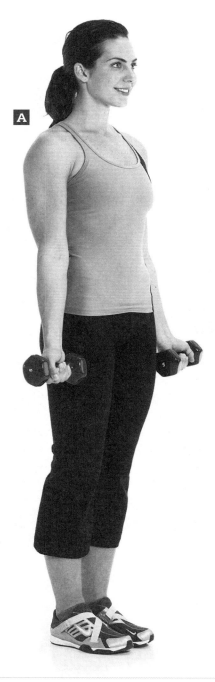

MAIN MOVE

A. Stand with feet together, holding a dumbbell in each hand, arms down at sides, palms facing forward.

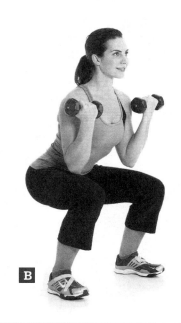

B. Step right foot about 2 feet out to side and bend knees and hips as if you were sitting back into a chair. Sit back as far as possible, keeping knees behind toes. At the same time, bend elbows, curling dumbbells up toward shoulders. Don't move upper arms or shoulders. As you stand back up, bring feet together and lower dumbbells. Complete one set, and then repeat, stepping to side with left foot.

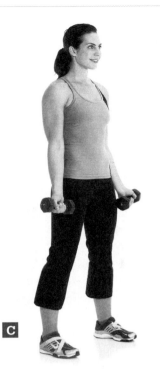

MAKE IT EASIER

C. Start with feet about shoulder-width apart and maintain this position as you do squats, without stepping to the side.

MAKE IT HARDER

D. As you stand back up from the squat position, raise left knee, bringing it in front of you to hip height, leg bent 90 degrees. Hold for 1 second, balancing on right foot, then swing left foot out to side and repeat. Complete one set, then repeat with opposite leg.

Side Lunge & Raise

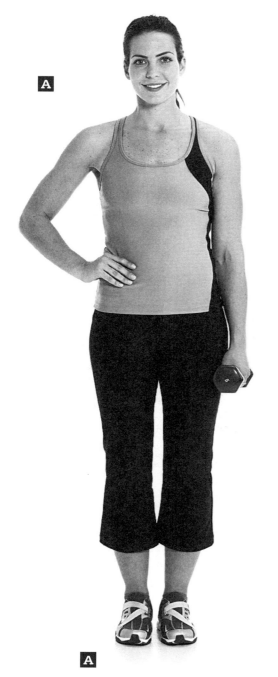

A

A

MAIN MOVE

A. Stand with feet together and hold a dumbbell in left hand with arm at side, palm facing in. Place right hand on hip.

B. Step right foot 2 to 3 feet out to side and bend right knee into a lunge, sitting back and bringing dumbbell toward right ankle. Keep right knee behind toes. Press off right foot and stand back up, bringing feet together. From this position, raise left arm out to left side until it's at shoulder height, and lift right leg out to opposite side, as high as possible (like photo at right). Hold for a second, then return to start position. Complete one set, then switch sides and repeat.

B

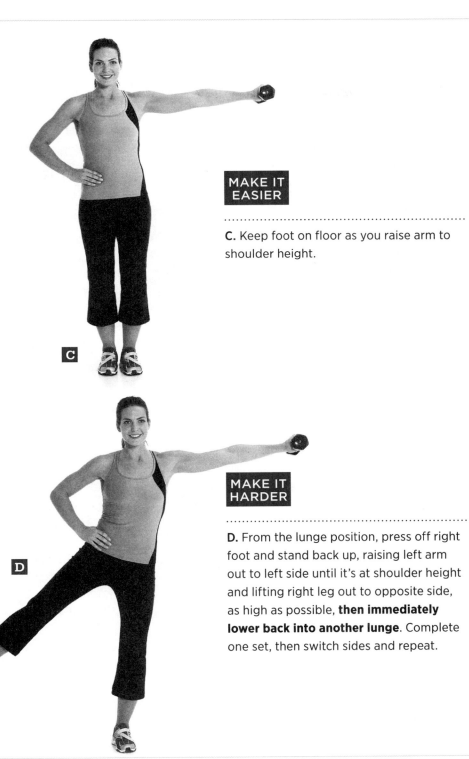

MAKE IT EASIER

....

C. Keep foot on floor as you raise arm to shoulder height.

MAKE IT HARDER

....

D. From the lunge position, press off right foot and stand back up, raising left arm out to left side until it's at shoulder height and lifting right leg out to opposite side, as high as possible, **then immediately lower back into another lunge**. Complete one set, then switch sides and repeat.

Pushup Row

A. Holding a dumbbell in each hand, get down on hands and knees. Walk hands forward so body forms a straight line from head to knees, and hands are directly beneath shoulders and feet are in the air.

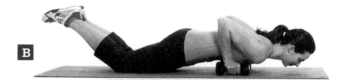

B. Bend elbows out to sides, lowering chest almost to floor. Press into hands, straightening arms back to start position. **C.** Then bend right elbow back, pulling dumbbell toward chest, keeping arm close to body. Lower dumbbell back to floor, and repeat from beginning, this time doing a row with left arm. Continue alternating rows for a full set, doing an extra rep each time so you do an equal number of rows with each arm.

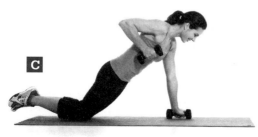

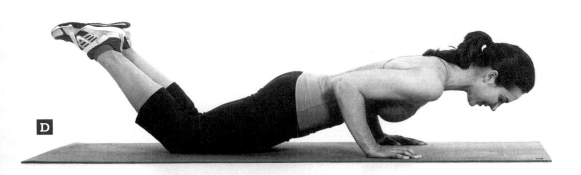

MAKE IT EASIER

Break up the moves. Do one set of pushups without dumbbells. **D.** Then get on hands and knees and do a set of rows with each arm.

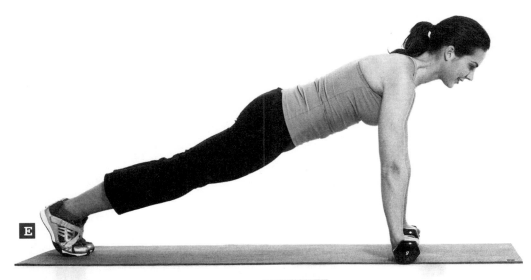

MAKE IT HARDER

E. Do full pushups, balancing on hands and toes.

The Belly Routine: Carve Those Abs

PART 3 OF the *Flat Belly* Workout focuses, of course, on your ab muscles. But I have another confession to make: When I was younger, I often skipped those last 5 minutes of my step class that were devoted to ab exercises for one reason: They consisted solely of crunches. *Bo-ring.* Plus they never seemed to do much for my middle. Our belly-toning workout is a combo routine that includes Pilates, traditional ab moves, and balance exercises to ensure that you're toning your midsection from every angle. All of these moves have been lab-tested and are guaranteed to deliver better results than ordinary crunches.

The roll-up works the main belly muscle, the rectus abdominis, which runs from the bottom of your ribs down to your pelvis, and is 80 percent more effective than a standard crunch.

The bicycle move is our pick if you only have time for one exercise. It targets the main ab muscle more effectively while also working your obliques, the muscles that wrap around your torso. This generates 190 percent more activity than when you do a simple crunch, according to an American Council on Exercise study.

Moves like the plank and arm and leg extension work both your abdominal and back muscles at the same time. Strong back muscles allow you to stand taller,

Stretch Your Workout Benefits

The most important thing you can do before exercise is to warm up with gentle activity. The best time to stretch is postworkout, when your muscles are warm and pliable. Stretching then also helps promote recovery and will improve your posture so you stand taller, making your belly look flatter instantly.

These three stretches target the major muscle groups that you'll be working. Gently ease in and out of the stretches,

holding each for 10 seconds. Don't bounce. Do each stretch three to six times, taking deep breaths throughout.

■ QUAD STRETCH Standing with feet together, bend left leg behind you, bringing that foot toward buttocks. (You can hold on to a chair or wall with right hand for balance if needed.) Grasp left foot with left hand and tuck hips under so you feel a stretch in the

improving posture—bonus—and helping your belly look flatter almost instantly.

Finally, the pike zeros in on those lower abs. Since the rectus abdominis is one long, continuous muscle, you can't completely isolate your upper and lower abs. But this exercise allows you to maximize the amount of work that the muscle fibers in the lower portion of that muscle are doing, activating it more than regular crunches, while also stimulating the upper portion.

Bottom line? Not a crunch in the bunch. And now you know why.

THE BELLY ROUTINE WEEKLY PLAN

WEEK	DAY 1	DAY 3	DAY 5
1	10 reps	10 reps	10 reps
2	15 reps	15 reps	15 reps
3	2 sets, 10 reps	2 sets, 10 reps	2 sets, 10 reps
4	2 sets, 15 reps	2 sets, 15 reps	2 sets, 15 reps

front of left thigh and hip. Hold for 10 seconds and release. Switch legs and repeat.

■ CALF STRETCH Stand with right foot about 2 to 3 feet in front of left, toes pointing forward. Place hands on right thigh and bend right knee, keeping left leg straight and pressing left heel into floor so you feel a stretch in left calf. Hold for 10 seconds and release. Switch legs and repeat.

■ HAMSTRING STRETCH From the calf stretch position, step back foot in 6 to 12 inches. Straighten front leg, lifting front toes off floor, and bend back leg and sit back, placing hands on thigh. It is very important not to lock your front knee. You should feel a stretch down the back of the thigh of your straight leg. Hold for 10 seconds and release. Switch legs and repeat.

Bicycle

A. Lie faceup with knees above hips, calves parallel to floor, and hands behind head.

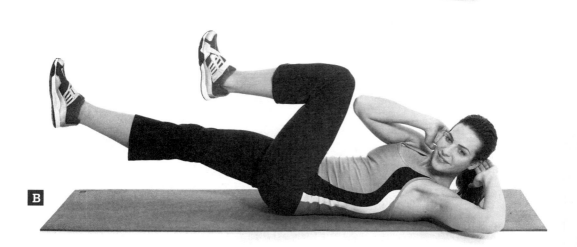

B. Contract abs, raising head and shoulders off floor as you extend right leg so it's about 10 inches off floor. Twist to left, bringing right elbow and left knee toward each other. Don't pull on your neck; the work should come from your abs. Hold for a second, then switch sides, twisting to right. That's one rep.

C. Keep feet flat on floor with knees bent as you lift and twist upper body.

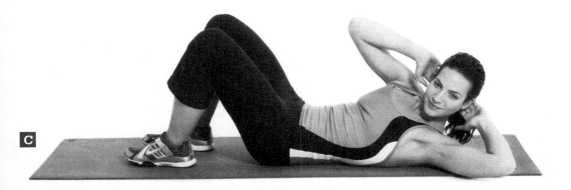

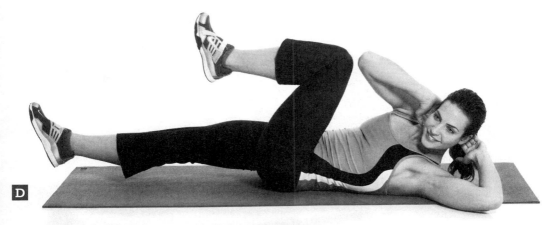

**MAKE IT
HARDER**

D. Lower extended leg farther so it's about 3 inches off floor.

Hover

A. Lie facedown with upper body propped on forearms and elbows directly beneath shoulders. Toes are tucked.

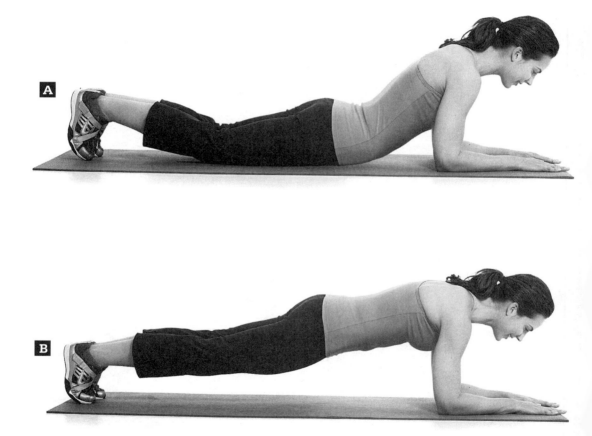

B. Contract torso muscles, lifting belly and legs off floor so body forms a straight line from head to heels. Keep abs tight so belly doesn't droop. Hold for 15 seconds (increase by 15 seconds each week so that by week 4 you're holding for 1 minute). One rep is all you need to do.

MAKE IT EASIER

....

C. Keep knees on floor and just lift belly, balancing on knees and forearms. Stay in this position.

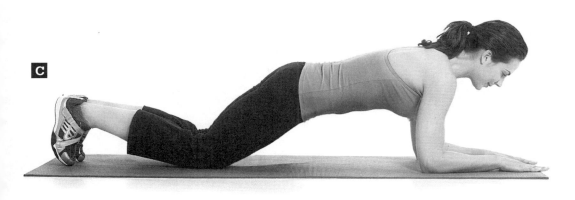

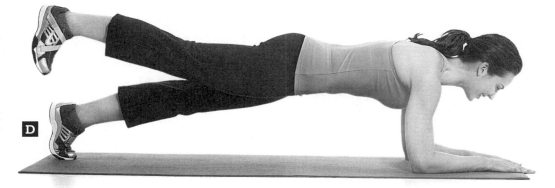

MAKE IT HARDER

....

D. Raise right foot off floor and hold for half the time, then switch legs and hold for remaining time.

Roll-Up

MAIN MOVE

A. Lie on back with arms extended overhead and legs bent, feet flat on floor.

B. Inhale and raise arms over chest. Then exhale and roll head toward chest, lifting head and shoulders off floor. (Keep arms next to ears throughout the move.) Press inner thighs together and pull navel in toward spine. Slowly peel off floor until you're sitting up.

Then extend legs so you're in a C shape—back rounded, head toward knees, and arms extended in front of you. Gradually reverse the movement, inhaling and squeezing abs as you roll back down to floor, one vertebra at a time.

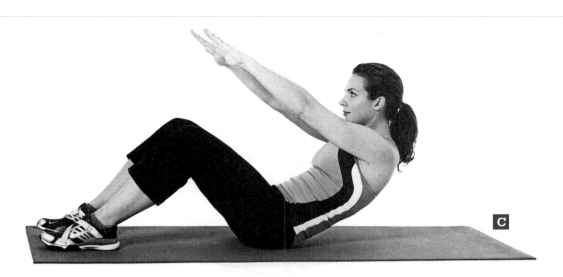

C

MAKE IT EASIER

....

C. Sit upright on floor with knees bent, feet flat, and arms extended at shoulder height in front of you. As you exhale, roll back only about 45 degrees, one vertebra at a time, keeping abs tight. Then roll back up.

MAKE IT HARDER

....

D. Do the move with legs extended the entire time.

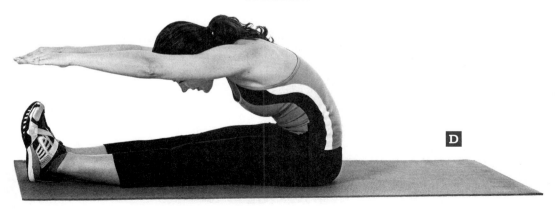

D

Arm & Leg Extension

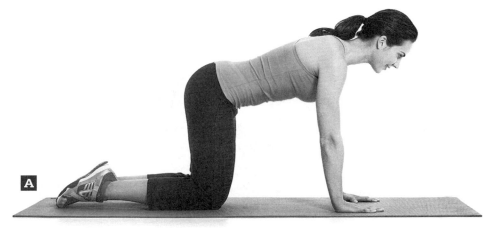

A

A. Kneel with hands directly beneath shoulders, and knees directly beneath hips.

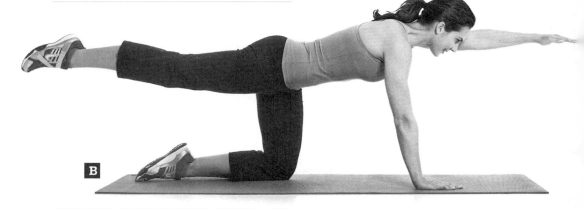

B

B. Keeping back straight and head in line with spine, simultaneously raise left arm and right leg, extending them in line with back so fingers are pointing straight ahead and toes are pointing behind you. Hold for a second, then lower. Perform one set, then switch arms and legs and repeat.

MAKE IT EASIER

C. Instead of lifting and lowering arm and leg, hold them in line with back for 15 seconds, then repeat on opposite side. One rep on each side is enough. Increase the amount of time you hold the move until you can do it for a full minute.

C

MAKE IT HARDER

D. When arm and leg are raised, contract abs and draw left elbow and right knee together beneath torso, holding for a second. Extend and repeat. Perform one set, then switch arms and legs and repeat.

Ab Pike

A. Lie faceup with arms at sides. Bend legs so feet are off floor, thighs over hips.

B. As you pull abs toward spine, lift hips up off floor, keeping legs bent. Keep hands and arms relaxed so you don't use them to help lift. Hold for a second, then slowly lower hips to floor and bend legs.

A

B

C. Lie with legs bent, feet flat on floor.
Contract abs, pressing small of back into
floor and curl hips up, doing a pelvic tilt,
without lifting feet.

MAKE IT
HARDER

D. As you lift hips, extend legs, and then
bend them as you lower.

PUTTING IT ALL TOGETHER: YOUR 28-DAY FLAT BELLY WORKOUT PLAN

WEEK	DAY 1	DAY 2	DAY 3	
1	Fat Blast Walk 30 min	Calorie Torch Walk 25 min	Fat Blast Walk 30 min	
	The Belly Routine 10 reps	The Metabolism Boost 10 reps	The Belly Routine 10 reps	
2	Fat Blast Walk 45 min	Calorie Torch Walk 35 min	Fat Blast Walk 45 min	
	The Belly Routine 15 reps	The Metabolism Boost 15 reps	The Belly Routine 15 reps	
3	Fat Blast Walk 60 min	Calorie Torch Walk 45 min	Fat Blast Walk 60 min	
	The Belly Routine 2 sets, 10 reps	The Metabolism Boost 2 sets, 10 reps	The Belly Routine 2 sets, 10 reps	
4	Fat Blast Walk 60 min	Calorie Torch Walk 45 min	Fat Blast Walk 60 min	
	The Belly Routine 2 sets, 15 reps	The Metabolism Boost 2 sets, 15 reps	The Belly Routine 2 sets, 15 reps	

DAY 4	DAY 5	DAY 6	DAY 7
Calorie Torch Walk 25 min	Fat Blast Walk 30 min	Calorie Torch Walk 25 min	REST
The Metabolism Boost 10 reps	The Belly Routine 10 reps	The Metabolism Boost 10 reps	
Calorie Torch Walk 35 min	Fat Blast Walk 45 min	Calorie Torch Walk 35 min	REST
The Metabolism Boost 15 reps	The Belly Routine 15 reps	The Metabolism Boost 15 reps	
Calorie Torch Walk 45 min	Fat Blast Walk 60 min	Calorie Torch Walk 45 min	REST
The Metabolism Boost 2 sets, 10 reps	The Belly Routine 2 sets, 10 reps	The Metabolism Boost 2 sets, 10 reps	
Calorie Torch Walk 45 min	Fat Blast Walk 60 min	Calorie Torch Walk 45 min	REST
The Metabolism Boost 2 sets, 15 reps	The Belly Routine 2 sets, 15 reps	The Metabolism Boost 2 sets, 15 reps	

Staying Motivated

AND NOW, A word about attitude. By now, you get it. Believing in yourself is integral to this entire Flat Belly journey. I see the power of attitude firsthand in every weight loss success story I edit at *Prevention* magazine and every time I meet a reader who's faced a life challenge head-on. The right outlook and perspective is what I always call the "special sauce." It means better results, faster results, and results that last.

I urge you to keep this in mind when the going gets rough: Changing your thought process can change your whole workout experience. In fact, your mind is so powerful that it can strengthen muscles without lifting a single dumbbell. When researchers at the Cleveland Clinic had healthy volunteers imagine that they were contracting the muscles in their hands, they increased hand strength by 35 percent. While this field of study is just beginning, imagine what your mind can do during an actual workout.

4 Reasons to Work Out to Music

1. You'll feel happier. A groundbreaking brain-imaging study from McGill University showed for the first time that music activates the same reward or pleasure centers in the brain that respond to the good feelings associated with eating and—believe it or not—sex.[5]

2. You'll move faster. Australian researchers discovered that the faster the beat, the more vigorously you work out. Other research has shown that exercisers who listen to music have more endurance and thus exercise longer, burning more calories.

3. You'll get smarter. In the first study to look at the combined effects of music and exercise on mental performance, Charles Emery, the study's lead author and a professor of psychology at Ohio State University, found that this duo increased scores on a verbal fluency test.[6]

4. You'll lose belly fat faster. Women who exercised to music lost as much as 8 pounds more than women who broke a sweat in silence.

Now, armed with this information, head into every workout imagining yourself strong, energized, and light as a feather. Don't recall moments from your tough day or dwell on how tired you feel. Instead, imagine yourself walking on clouds or that an invisible force is lifting you up, helping you take that next step, lift that weight, or complete that move. Your mind is a powerful thing. Use it! If you take just a few seconds to adjust your attitude, you won't believe how much easier, faster, and enjoyable your workout will be.

What if I'm an avid exerciser? Should I stick with my regular routine or do this routine?

If you have an exercise program you love, absolutely keep it up. You're more likely to stick with exercise if you're doing something you enjoy. But I would encourage you to compare your workouts to those recommended here, and maybe make some minor adjustments to your exercise plan to maximize its belly-flattening potential. Here are some questions to ask yourself as you review your plan.

■ *Am I lifting weights at least 2 days a week?*
If not, consider adding **The Metabolism Boost** moves on pages 288 to 295 to your workout schedule. If you are but want to see better results, aim for 3 days a week of strength training, working in some of the combo moves from **The Metabolism Boost**. By working multiple body parts at the same time, you'll burn more calories.

■ *Am I doing 30 to 60 minutes of cardio exercise (walking, biking, jogging, swimming, using a cardio machine like an elliptical or stairclimber) at least 5 days a week?*
If not, increase the length or frequency of your workouts to boost your daily calorie burn. If you are but want to see better results, turn three of your sessions into interval workouts—like the **Calorie Torch** walk. Or, turn any cardio activity into an interval routine by increasing the intensity for 30 to 60 seconds and then slowing down to your usual pace for 2 to 5 minutes.

■ *Am I doing any belly-focused exercises at least 2 days a week?*
If not, start by just doing one or two moves from **The Belly Routine** on pages 298 to 307 per session to firm up your midsection.

READ A FLAT BELLY
SUCCESS
STORY

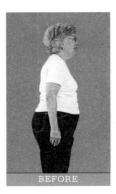

BEFORE

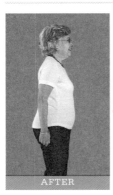

AFTER

Evelyn Gomer

POUNDS LOST:

7

IN 32 DAYS

ALL-OVER INCHES LOST:

8.5

EVELYN GOMER'S MOTIVATION TO TRY THE *FLAT BELLY DIET* came from her friends—Indirectly, anyway. "For years, I was a city person—New York City, that is. Most city women are skinny and dress beautifully, and that was me for years—until I moved away from Manhattan." As Evelyn tells it, "I married late in life and moved to the suburbs, where the women were more, well, matronly. So for whatever reason, I just let myself go—completely." She and her husband moved back to New York, and she found her city friends were still skinny and svelte—but she wasn't. "I wanted to get back into that," she says. "So when I heard about this diet, I jumped at the chance to try it." It's not that she hadn't dieted before. She had—but not with any lasting success. "This one? What a blessing!"

The first really wonderful thing she found was that she was never hungry. "I'm very uncomfortable when I'm hungry. My stomach growls, and I get very tired and listless. But eating the four meals a day worked for me. And those MUFAs!" Like most of the Flat Belly dieters, Evelyn had never heard of a MUFA before being introduced to the diet, so when she heard she could have nuts, she was happier than happy. "I adore nuts—all kinds. They actually helped alleviate any yen for richer desserts. I still can't believe that something so fattening can be so healthy," she says. "I travel with a jar of peanut butter just in case I'm not in a place where I can find what I want to eat. I can be satisfied just nibbling on nuts. But there are so many other wonderful things to choose from, too."

Evelyn is all about convenience. She read the 28 days of meals and recipes and selected about 20 meals that she could be happy with and that didn't require "50 million ingredients." She's been making those same meals over and over. She says that after a while you get to know them by heart and you don't have to read what you need. You do a major shop, and you have all the ingredients in the house.

She brings up an additional benefit she has seen from the *Flat Belly Diet,* one in addition to her 7 pounds and 8.5 inches lost over 4 weeks. It seems her husband is getting thinner, too. "No," she says, "he's not on the diet. It's just that I haven't been cooking much, so he's fending for himself and eating a lot less than he usually eats. He's lost weight, and he's very happy about that."

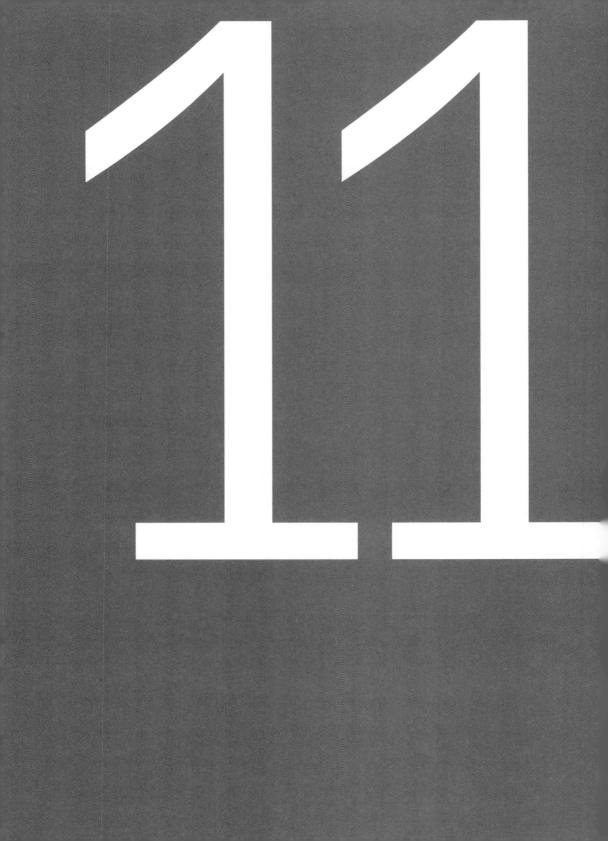

YOUR GUIDE TO
DAY 33
AND BEYOND

HERE ARE TWO revealing statistics: On the one hand, a recent survey found that the percentage of people dieting to lose weight at any given time has fallen to 29 percent, down from 33 percent in 2004.[1] Yet, on the other hand, people are beginning to eat healthier in growing, even stunning, numbers. Fifty-seven percent of shoppers are trying to eat healthfully, up from 45 percent in 2000.[2]

Americans are eating more fruits and vegetables and whole grains than we have in the past, and in some surveys as many as 90 percent are doing something to improve the healthfulness of their meals, like limiting salt, sugar, or saturated fat or paying more attention to portions. That says to me that people are more interested in making food choices that impact their long-term health than they are in following some gimmicky, quick-fix plan. That's why I wanted the *Flat Belly Diet* to be—first and foremost—something readers could sustain for the rest of their lives.

So, here we are. You've presumably finished the first 32 days of the *Flat Belly Diet*, so let's take a look back at what you've achieved. If you've followed the parameters of this plan (eating your MUFAs at every meal, limiting calories to 1,600 a day, exercising on a regular basis in a smart, efficient way, and coming to a deeper realization about how you think about food), then you've taken the first and most difficult step toward a healthier future. And—nice bonus here—you've most likely lost a few pounds of the deadliest fat you can have: belly fat.

I also hope you've learned a few things that will make living the *Flat Belly Diet* lifestyle even more rewarding. You know the anatomy and physiology of the digestive system better than ever before. You understand why the fat you can't see is sometimes scarier than the fat that pokes out over your jeans. And you've read about the intricate connection between stress, cortisol, and your body. Putting all this knowledge to work for you, your belly, and your health in an ongoing way is as simple as permanently adopting the three *Flat Belly Diet* rules that are probably quite familiar to you by now. I hope you've discovered that it really is possible to follow the *Flat Belly Diet* forever.

Our test panelists certainly did. After ending the test phase of the *Flat Belly Diet*, every single one, without being asked, said they planned to stick with the program. Why? Because they lost weight and inches and never felt deprived. Because week after week they reported no hunger, energy through the roof, and no cravings. They gave the meals and recipes rave reviews. And they loved knowing that once they understood the plan, they didn't have to count the days until they could eat satisfying meals again.

Remember, succeeding on the *Flat Belly Diet* promises an even greater reward than a visually attractive silhouette: It promises a longer, healthier life. This chapter is all about getting you fully armed to reap *all* the rewards of the *Flat Belly Diet*—flat belly included—for decades to come.

Flat Belly for Life: Rules to Eat By

- **Rule #1** Stick to 400 calories per meal.

- **Rule #2** Never go more than 4 hours without eating.

- **Rule #3** Eat a MUFA at every meal.

RULE #1: STICK TO 400 CALORIES PER MEAL.

I'M NOT GOING to mince words here: To keep your weight down and your metabolism on track, you must continue to control your daily caloric intake— that is, stick to about 400 calories per meal, 1,600 per day. Why, you're wondering, do you have to maintain the same daily calorie intake that got you to your goal, *after* you've reached that goal? Because the fact of the matter is, 1,600 calories is enough to keep up your energy, support your immune system, and maintain your precious calorie-burning muscle (so you won't feel run-down, cranky, or hungry), but it's not enough calories to allow you to gain back your belly fat (and make you more vulnerable to all the attendant health risks).

I am in no way sentencing you to a life of deprivation or boredom here. You've been eating the *Flat Belly Diet* way for 32 days, and you know firsthand how satisfying and hunger free this lifestyle is. One of the main reasons the *Flat Belly Diet* worked for you is that the food is nothing less than fabulous. And there's no shortage of it. And boredom? Forget about it. Between the quick-fix meals, Snack Packs, and recipes, as well as a multitude of approved packaged and fast food items, you have hundreds of choices, whether or not you have the time (or the inclination) to cook.

RULE #2: NEVER GO MORE THAN 4 HOURS WITHOUT EATING.

THIS IS YOUR tried-and-true routine by now. You've established a rhythm, and your body has responded—by becoming accustomed to having three MUFA-rich 400-calorie meals at 4-hour intervals, as well as a healthy Snack Pack at whatever time of day suits you. You now know how it feels to keep your energy up, your blood sugar steady, your metabolism revved—what it's like to have control of your appetite. And you've seen the results, belly-wise. Stick with it and it will continue to benefit your health and your waistline.

RULE #3: EAT A MUFA AT EVERY MEAL.

OVER THE PAST few weeks, you have come to know MUFAs well (and love them as dearly as I do, I'm sure!), those little miracle workers in your belly that help you feel full *and* lose visceral fat from your middle. You've also discovered how easy—and tasty—it is to include small amounts of these healthy fats in your meals. Even if you can't work in a MUFA at every single meal you ever eat, you know that they are found mainly in vegetable oils, nuts, seeds, olives, and avocados. They are about as easy to come by as they are to love, and it won't be difficult for you to put the MUFA rule into practice most of the time. And if you don't know the MUFA list by heart at this point, you can always flip to page 101 for a quick reference.

A Flat Belly for Life: Strategies to Live By

TIME AND AGAIN throughout this book I've told you, the Flat Belly Diet is about *attitude*. Well, guess what—so is your healthy, flat-bellied future.

I've supplied you with tools and tricks galore that, as you move forward beyond Day 32, are going to be no less important to nourishing and fortifying you than the *Flat Belly* meals and MUFAs. These tools and tricks have been as integral to your success as the foods you've eaten. You've used them to make major changes. And they'll be just as essential to your ongoing health and well-being.

I've boiled it down to a few key practices and pointers. Use these as a guide for in your journey ahead.

KEEP JOURNALING

As I NOTED in Chapter 9, journaling is probably the single most important thing you can do going forward to help you maintain your focus on your long-term health goals. Trust me when I say it will help you stay on track. I'm not suggesting that you write something for 15 minutes every day for the rest of your life. I am, however, urging you to keep a journal in your repertoire of health tools. Just as no parent should be without a thermometer in the medicine cabinet, I firmly believe that no woman should be without the means to record her thoughts and feelings on paper (or on a computer). Your journal is your emotional thermometer. Your thoughts are the clues to all your destruc-

The Danger of Skipping Meals

It doesn't pay to try to dip below the 1,600-calories-a-day mark. Believe me, I understand the temptation. We've all been led to believe that the fewer calories we ingest, the faster we'll drop the pounds. But weight loss isn't quite that simple. If you drastically cut down on the amount of food you eat for any extended period of time, your body's natural response is to slow things down in order to conserve fat. For those of us who aspire to flatter bellies, that "starvation response" is the last thing we need.

Here's what happens: If you take in too few calories, your body starts breaking down muscle tissue to use for fuel. That muscle loss can drastically affect your metabolism, often for long periods of time. The reason is simple: Muscle is metaboli-

cally active tissue that requires a certain number of calories each day to maintain itself, whether or not it's in use. So the more muscle you have, the more calories you burn. As your muscle mass drops, so does your body's need for calories to sustain it. Let's say a dieter on a too-strict plan loses 15 pounds—10 of which is fat and 5 of which is muscle. Let's also assume that every pound of muscle burns about 50 calories a day. With this muscle tissue gone, the dieter must now consume 250 (5 times 50) fewer calories a day in order to *maintain* her 15-pound weight loss.

Of course, most dieters don't stick with the strict routine for long; they return to their prediet eating habits. And that's what puts them at risk of regaining all their lost weight—and then some.

tive insecurities and all your inner power. Why on earth would you consider ignoring them?

STAY MINDFUL

Whenever you need a quick attitude adjustment from frantic to focused, call on the Mind Tricks from Chapter 5. They're fast—just minutes apiece—but

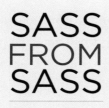

SASS FROM SASS

"Avoid These Common Pitfalls"

As a dietitian, I've helped hundreds of people lose weight, but I've also lived with a successful "loser" for over a decade. Seeing my husband, Jack, shed more than 50 pounds and never gain it back has shown me firsthand that, while it's not always easy, it is possible to lose a significant amount of weight *and* keep it off. A recent study looked at the key reasons why successful losers so often regain the weight they've lost. I can say that Jack's a pro at avoiding each one of these pitfalls, and you can be, too.

Pitfall #1: failing to plan in advance before social situations. Prevent it by bringing your own meals or snacks when you're going to hang out with friends or family, or host get-togethers at your place so you have more control over the menu.

Pitfall #2: feeling deprived. According to our testers, this wasn't an issue on the *Flat Belly Diet*. Over and over we heard that they didn't feel deprived at all and even felt a little guilty about how full and satisfied they were. That's because the food on this plan is delicious and includes healthy indulgences like chocolate, nuts, cheese, and berries.

Pitfall #3: underestimating the number of calories in foods. We've made this one a no-brainer. The *Flat Belly Diet* controls your calories for you so you can't go overboard.

—*Cynthia*

extremely effective at jolting you out of a stress-fueled stupor and adjusting your emotional relationship to eating. They'll help you slow down, take your time, and savor your meals, so you won't be tempted to overindulge or eat too quickly.

MANAGE STRESS

THE STRESS/BELLY FAT connection is clear. Manage stress and you are one step closer to managing your belly fat forever. Writing in your journal can be a great stress reliever, but so can daily exercise. (Another reason that I like to walk to and from work is that I get to work out solutions to office crises in my head, entertaining passersby by occasionally talking to myself.) If you need more ideas to help get your stress under control, periodically revisit the stress-busting strategies in Chapter 4 and use as a checklist.

GATHER A SUPPORT TEAM

ONE OF THE best ways to stay on track and stay motivated is to have a support team behind you. Regardless of how motivated you are, long-term success is always easier with help from others. Even one person will do—just someone to tell you you're doing great every once in a while. Having people in your life who understand and accept your dreams can make all the difference in the world. Your supporters don't have to be members of your family or even good friends, so long as they respect your goals.

Results in the Real World

SCALE NOT BUDGING? At a certain point, every dieter hits a plateau. Here's why it happens. The *Flat Belly Diet* is designed to only give you enough calories—1,600—to support a healthy, "ideal" weight. If you weigh more than your ideal weight, you are consuming more than 1,600 calories a day. You may jump up and down and tell me that no, you know for a fact that you're only eating 1,200 calories a day, you're starving, and you still don't lose weight. And I would say *hooey*. Just as you need a certain amount of wood to heat a log cabin, you need a certain amount of calories to keep yourself alive. And the more you weigh, the more calories you need to maintain that weight. Just by going on this plan, you've created a calorie deficit that will allow you to drop pounds. With every pound you lose, however, this calorie deficit shrinks, so as you get closer and closer to your weight goal, it takes longer and longer to lose the next pound.

It doesn't seem fair, but it's the laws of physics! On this plan, you should never hit a true plateau (that is, no net loss). But at times it might feel like your weight loss has stalled. If you're following the plan—and keeping a food journal—I can assure you it has not stalled. It has just slowed. Think about it like this—if you were losing 2 pounds a week, then just 1 pound a week, you'll eventually get to ½ pound a week, then ¼. Those incremental losses probably won't register on your scale, but a loss is still a loss. Remember that even ¼ pound of fat loss is a full stick of butter zapped from your body. That's still amazing progress in 1 week's time!

The Flat Belly Diet to Go:
The Angst-Free Guide to Dining Out

OKAY, YOU'VE GOT this gorgeous, flat belly, you're full of energy, and you feel absolutely wonderful. Now it's time to celebrate. Maybe it's your anniversary. Or your birthday. Or maybe you're just feeling happy. Dinner out? Why not?

Just remember, you are there to celebrate, not binge. And if you stay with the program—or even a slightly modified version—you will wake up feeling good, not guilty, tomorrow. Go ahead, treat yourself to something special. If you plan ahead, there's no reason why you shouldn't be able to enjoy a meal anywhere you want, and that includes pizza with your girlfriends after an afternoon of shopping at the mall. Following these guidelines will help you stay on track.

■ Eat what you would normally eat throughout the day. Skipping a meal in order to save calories for later just increases the chances that you will overeat at dinner. You can also up your exercise—the added calorie burn will help offset a splurge like dessert.

■ Have a light snack before you go out. Good options include *Flat Belly Diet* smoothies or anything that incudes a MUFA. The MUFA will take the edge off your hunger and help you pass up the bread basket.

■ Be the first at the table to order. This will keep you from being tempted by others' choices.

■ Try to leave some food on your plate. The old "clean plate" rules from childhood no longer apply.

Portion Patrol

PERHAPS THE MOST important tip for dining out is to watch the size of your portions. It goes without saying that anything called "super size" is something to be avoided, but beware dishes that don't advertise their generous proportions but provide enough for two or three people. It always helps to have a visual reference to help moderate your portions of different foods when dining out. For example:

DID YOU KNOW?

Research published in the *Journal of the American Medical Association* revealed that women who exercised 5 days per week for 30 to 45 minutes at a time for a full year were able to reduce belly fat by 3 to 6 percent.[7]

■ One-half cup of cooked rice or pasta is considered one "serving." This is about the size of a mini fruit cup or half a baseball. If you're trying to limit your portion of rice or pasta to two servings: Think two mini fruit cups or one baseball. Most Chinese restaurants provide far more than this amount of rice.

■ One standard-size slice of bread is considered one "serving" of bread. Compare rolls, buns, and other bread products to this mental image and adjust your portion size accordingly: If the bun on your chicken sandwich or burger looks larger than two slices of bread, leave some bread on the plate.

■ Three ounces of cooked meat, the size of a deck of cards or woman's palm, is considered one "serving." Most restaurants provide far more than this amount in an entrée. Savvy ways to cut back include ordering a half portion, having a sandwich instead of an entrée, or splitting a meal.

■ One-fourth cup of shredded cheese is considered a single portion. That's about the size of a golf ball. According to the 2005 Dietary Guidelines, healthy adults need two to three servings of milk, yogurt, or cheese per day. If cheese is your weakness, think "golf ball" the next time you sprinkle cheese on your food.

In Closing

I'D LIKE TO close by reminding you of the very last question I asked you in Chapter 4: *Who are you doing this for?* There is still only one acceptable answer to that question, whether you choose to continue with this plan one day at a time or enroll in the online service **flatbellydiet.com** for life. That answer is "*for me.*" If you weren't quite sure of that back then, I hope that with the Core Confidences in Chapter 9, I have given you the tools to arrive at that answer now.

This plan was created to help you see that focusing on yourself isn't an exercise in selfishness. In today's day and age, we are all overly committed to other people, whether it's the attention we lavish on our children and spouse, or the time we spend at our jobs, or the effort we put into building our communities. But I speak from experience when I tell you that none of those commitments is worth anything if you aren't first and foremost committed to yourself. The *Flat Belly Diet* is not a vanity ploy. Sure, it's a weight-loss plan designed to give you a sexier waistline. But it's not a crazy detox diet that promises you the abs of a 20-year-old. It is a weight-loss plan based on the most credible—and safe—science that targets the most dangerous type of fat you carry on your body, the fat that threatens your very existence. If you want to live longer and healthier, keeping that fat is simply not an option.

I hope that you will continue to eat the *Flat Belly Diet* way for as long as it takes for you to experience the freedom that comes from a healthier body weight. If you end up with abs of steel, I will be over-the-moon thrilled for you! (Although maybe just a teensy bit jealous.) But I'd be just as happy if you were to tell me that you finally lost your pregnancy weight, or you started walking or lowered your blood pressure, or you stopped buying shapeless, oversize tunics because you no longer feel self-conscious about the way you look. This plan is less about achieving an ideal body than it is about creating a healthier life. If you remember nothing about the *Flat Belly Diet* but the fact that a MUFA at every meal could save your life, then I've done my job. And you've done yours.

endnotes

Chapter 1

1. J.A. Paniagua, A. Gallego de la Sacristana, I. Romero, A. Vidal-Puig, J.M. Latre, E. Sanchez, P. Perez-Martinez, J. Lopez-Miranda, and F. Perez-Jimenez, "Monounsaturated Fat–Rich Diet Prevents Central Body Fat Distribution and Decreases Postprandial Adiponectin Expression Induced by a Carbohydrate-Rich Diet in Insulin-Resistant Subjects," *Diabetes Care*, 30 (2007):1717–23.

Chapter 2

1. R.E. Ostlund, M. Staten, W.M. Kohrt, J. Schultz, and M. Malley, "The Ratio of Waist-to-Hip Circumference, Plasma Insulin Level, and Glucose Intolerance as Independent Predictors of the HDL2 Cholesterol Level in Older Adults," *New England Journal of Medicine*, 322, no. 4 (January 25, 1990):229–34.
2. László B. Tankó, Yu Z. Bagger, Peter Alexandersen, Philip J. Larsen, Claus Christiansen, "Peripheral Adiposity Exhibits an Independent Dominant Antiatherogenic Effect in Elderly Women," *Circulation*, 107 (2003):1626.
3. Frank B. Hu; Tricia Y. Li; Graham A. Colditz; Walter C. Willett; JoAnn E. Manson, "Television Watching and Other Sedentary Behaviors in Relation to Risk of Obesity and Type 2 Diabetes Mellitus in Women," *JAMA*, 289 (2003):1785–91.
4. R.A. Whitmer, S. Sidney, J. Selby, S. Claiborne Johnston, and K. Yaffe, "Midlife Cardiovascular Risk Factors and Risk of Dementia in Late Life," *Neurology*, 64 (2005):277–81.
5. http://win.niddk.nih.gov/publications/tools.htm#circumf.
6. http://www.rush.edu/itools/hip/hipcalc.html.
7. "Thin People May Be Obese on the Inside," *Medical Research News*, May 14, 2007, reporting a study funded by the Medical Research Council under the direction of Dr. Jimmy Bell, professor of molecular imaging at Imperial College, London, http://www.news-medical.net/?id=25076.
8. Salim Yusuf, Steven Hawken, et al. "Obesity and the Risk of Myocardial Infarction in 27,000 Participants from 52 Countries; A Case-Control Study," *Lancet*, 366 (2005):1640–49.
9. "Modest Gain in Visceral Fat Causes Dysfunction of Blood Vessel Lining in Lean Healthy Humans; Shedding Weight Restores Vessel Health," presented by the Mayo Clinic team at the American Heart Association's Scientific Sessions, November 2007, http://www.sciencedaily.com/releases/2007/11/071105121934.htm.

Chapter 3

1. S. J. Nicholls, P. Lundman, J. A. Harmer, B. Cutri, K. A. Griffiths, K. A. Rye, P. J. Barter, and D. S. Celermajer, "Consumption of Saturated Fat Impairs the Anti-inflammatory Properties of High-Density Lipoproteins and Endothelial Function," *Journal of the American College of Cardiology*, 48, no. 4 (2006):715–20.

2. David Kritchevsky, "History of Recommendations to the Public about Dietary Fat," *The Journal of Nutrition*, 128, no. 2 (1998):449S–452S.

3. U.S. Department of Health and Human Services and U.S. Department of Agriculture, "Nutrition and Your Health: Dietary Guidelines for Americans, 1980," http://www.health.gov/dietaryguidelines/1980thin.pdf.

4. U.S. Department of Health and Human Services and U.S. Department of Agriculture, "Nutrition and Your Health: Dietary Guidelines for Americans, 1995," http://www.health.gov/dietaryguidelines/dga95/default.htm.

5. U.S. Department of Health and Human Services and U.S. Department of Agriculture, "Nutrition and Your Health: Dietary Guidelines for Americans, 2000," http://www.health.gov/dietaryguidelines/dga2000/document/frontcover.htm.

6. U.S. Department of Health and Human Services and U.S. Department of Agriculture, "Dietary Guidelines for Americans, 2005," http://www.health.gov/dietaryguidelines/dga2005/document/default.htm.

7. T. Thom, N. Haase, W. Rosamond, V. J. Howard, J. Rumsfeld, T. Manolio, Z. J. Zheng, K. Flegal, C. O'Donnell, S. Kittner, D. Lloyd-Jones, D. C. Goff Jr., Y. Hong, R. Adams, G. Friday, K. Furie, P. Gorelick, B. Kissela, J. Marler, J. Meigs, V. Roger, S. Sidney, P. Sorlie, J. Steinberger, S. Wasserthiel-Smoller, M. Wilson, and P. Wolf, American Heart Association Statistics Committee and Stroke Statistics Subcommittee, "Heart Disease and Stroke Statistics—2006 Update: A Report from the American Heart Association Statistics Committee and Stroke Statistics Subcommittee," *Circulation*, 113, no. 6 (2006):e85–151.

8. National Center for Health Statistics, "National Health and Nutrition Examination Survey," http://www.cdc.gov/nchs/about/major/nhanes/nh1rrm.htm.

9. A. Keys, C. Aravanis, H. W. Blackburn, F. S. Van Buchem, R. Buzina, B. D. Djordjevic, A. S. Dontas, F. Fidanza, M. J. Karvonen, N. Kimura, D. Lekos, M. Monti, V. Puddu, and H. L Taylor, "Epidemiological Studies Related to Coronary Heart Disease: Characteristics of Men Aged 40–59 in Seven Countries," *Acta Medica Scandinavica Supplementum*, 460 (1966):1–392.

10. M. D. Kontogianni, D. B. Panagiotakos, C. Chrysohoou, C. Pitsavos, A. Zampelas, and C. Stefanadis, "The Impact of Olive Oil Consumption Pattern on the Risk of Actute Coronary Syndromes: The CARDIO2000 Case-Control Study," *Clinical Cardiology*, 30, no. 3 (2007):125–9.

11. H. M. Roche, A. Zampelas, J. M. Knapper, D. Webb, C. Brooks, K. G. Jackson, J. W. Wright, B. J. Gould, A. Kafatos, M. J. Gibney, and C. M. Williams, "Effect of Long-

Term Olive Oil Dietary Intervention on Postprandial Triacylglycerol and Factor VII Metabolism," *American Journal of Clinical Nutrition*, 68, no. 3 (1998):552–60.

12. W. R. Archer, B. Lamarche, A. C. St-Pierre, J. F. Mauger, O. Deriaz, N. Landry, L. Corneau, J. P. Despres, J. Bergeron, J. Couture, and N. Bergeron, "High Carbohydrate and High Monounsaturated Fatty Acid Diets Similarly Affect LDL Electrophoretic Characteristics in Men Who Are Losing Weight," *Journal of Nutrition*, 133, no. 10 (2003):3124–9.

13. L. J. Appel, F. M. Sacks, V. J. Carey, E. Obarzanek, J. F. Swain, E. R. Miller III, P. R. Conlin, T. P. Erlinger, B. A. Rosner, N. M. Laranjo, J. Charleston, P. McCarron, and L. M. Bishop, OmniHeart Collaborative Research Group, "Effects of Protein, Monounsaturated Fat, and Carbohydrate Intake on Blood Pressure and Serum Lipids: Results of the Omniheart Randomized Trial," *The Journal of the American Medical Association*, 294, no. 19 (2005):2455–64.

14. P. M. Kris-Etherton, T. A. Pearson, Y. Wan, R. L. Hargrove, K. Moriarty, V. Fishell, and T. D. Etherton, "High-Monounsaturated Fatty Acid Diets Lower Both Plasma Cholesterol and Triacylglycerol Concentrations," *American Journal of Clinical Nutrition*, 70, no. 6 (1999):1009–15.

15. R. Estruch, M. A. Martinez-Gonzalez, D. Corella, J. Salas-Salvado, V. Ruiz-Gutierrez, M. I. Covas, M. Fiol, E. Gomez-Gracia, M. C. Lopez-Sabater, E. Vinyoles, F. Aros, M. Conde, C. Hahoz, J. Lapetra, G. Saez, and E. Ros, PREDIMED Study Investigators, "Effects of a Mediterranean-Style Diet on Cardiovascular Risk Factors: A Randomized Trial," *Annals of Internal Medicine*, 145, no. 1 (2006):1–11.

16. National Institutes of Health, "How You Can Lower Your Cholesterol Level," http://www.nhlbi.nih.gov/chd/lifestyles.htm.

17. J. A. Paniagua, A. Gallego de la Sacristana, I. Romero, A. Vidal-Puig, J. M. Latre, E. Sanchez, P. Perez-Martinez, J. Lopez-Miranda, and F. Perez-Jimenez, "Monounsaturated Fat-Rich Diet Prevents Central Body Fat Distribution and Decreases Postprandial Adiponectin Expression Induced by a Carbohydrate-Rich Diet in Insulin-Resistant Subjects," *Diabetes Care*, 30, no. 7 (2007):1717–23.

18. B. Gumbiner, C. C. Low, and P. D. Reaven, "Effects of a Monounsaturated Fatty Acid-Enriched Hypocaloric Diet on Cardiovascular Risk Factors in Obese Patients with Type 2 Diabetes," *Diabetes Care*, 21, no. 1 (1998):9–15.

19. C. Romero, E. Medina, J. Vargas, M. Brenes, and A. De Castro, "In Vitro Activity of Olive Oil Polyphenols against *Helicobacter pylori*," *Journal of Agriculture and Food Chemistry,* 55, no. 3 (2007):680–686.

20. G. Zhao, T. D. Etherton, K. R. Martin, S. G. West, P. J. Gillies, and P. M. Kris-Etherton, "Dietary Alpha-Linolenic Acid Reduces Inflammatory and Lipid Cardiovascular Risk Factors in Hypercholesterolemic Men and Women," *Journal of Nutrition*, 134 (2004):2991–2997.

21. N. Z. Unlu, T. Bohn, S. K. Clinton, and S. J. Schwartz, "Carotenoid Absorption from Salad and Salsa by Humans Is Enhanced by the Addition of Avocado or Avocado Oil," *The Journal of Nutrition*, 135, no. 3 (2005):431–436.

22. L. Berglund, M. Lefebre, H. N. Ginsberg, P. M. Kris-Etherton, P. J. Elmer, P. W. Stewart, A. Ershow, T. A. Pearson, B. H. Dennis, P. S. Roheim, R. Ramakrishnan, R. Reed, K. Stewart, and K. M. Phillips, DELTA Investigators, "Comparison of Monounsaturated Fat with Carbohydrates as a Replacement for Saturated Fat in Subjects with a High Metabolic Risk Profile: Studies in the Fasting and Postprandial States," *American Journal of Clinical Nutrition*, 86, no. 6 (2007): 611–20.

23. J. Salas-Salvado, A. Garcia-Arellano, F. Estruch, F. Marquez-Sandoval, D. Corella, M. Fiol, E. Gomez-Gracia, E. Vinoles, F. Aros, C. Herrera, C. Lahoz, J. Lapetra, J. S. Perona, D. Munoz-Aguado, M. A. Martinez-Gonzalez, and E. Ros, "Components of the Mediterranean-Type Food Pattern and Serum Inflammatory Markers among Patients at High Risk for Cardiovascular Disease," *European Journal of Clinical Nutrition*, advance online publication doi: 10.1038/sj.ejcn.1602762 (18 April 2007), www.nature.com/ejcn/journal/vaop/ncurrent/abs/1602762a.html.

24. K. Esposito, R. Marfella, M. Ciotola, C. Di Palo, F. Giugliano, G. Fiugliano, M. D'Armiento, F. D'Andrea, and D. Giugliano, "Effect of a Mediterranean-Style Diet on Endothelial Dysfunction and Markers of Vascular Inflammation in the Metabolic Syndrome: A Randomized Trial," *The Journal of the American Medical Association*, 292, no. 12 (2004):1440–6.

25. A. Wolk, R. Bergstrom, D. Hunter, W. Willett, H. Ljung, L. Holmberg, L. Bergkvist, A. Bruce, and H. O. Adami, "A Prospective Study of Association of Monounsaturated Fat and Other Types of Fat with Risk of Breast Cancer," *Archives of Internal Medicine*, 158, no. 1 (1998):41–5.

26. V. Solfrizzi, F. Panza, F. Torres, F. Mastroianni, A. Del Parigi, A. Venezia, and A. Capurso, "High Monounsaturated Fatty Acids Intake Protects against Age-Related Cognitive Decline," *Neurology*, 52, no. 8 (1999):1563–9.

27. F. Panza, V. Solfrizzi, A. M. Colacicco, A. D'Introno, C. Capurso, F. Torres, A. Del Parigi, S. Capurso, and A. Capurso, "Mediterranean Diet and Cognitive Decline," *Public Health Nutrition*, 7, no. 7 (2004):959–63.

28. V. Solfrizzi, A. D'Introno, A. M. Colacicco, C. Capurso, R. Palasciano, S. Capurso, F. Torres, A. Capurso, and F. Panza, "Unsaturated Fatty Acids Intake and All-Causes Mortality: A 8.5-Year Follow-Up of the Italian Longitudinal Study on Aging," *Experimental Gerontology*, 40, no. 4 (2005):335–43.

29. J. A. Paniagua, A. Gallego dl la Sacristana, I. Romero, A. Vidal-Puig, J. M. Latre, E. Sanchez, P. Perez-Martinez, J. Lopez-Miranda, F. Perez-Jimenez, "Monounsaturated Fat-Rich Diet Prevents Central Body Fat Distribution and Decreases Postprandial Adiponectin Expression Induced by a Carbohydrate-Rich Diet in Insulin-Resistant Subjects," *Diabetes Care*, 3, no. 7 (2007):1717–23.

30. L. S. Piers, K. Z. Walker, R. M. Stoney, M. J. Soares, and K. O'Dea, "The Influence of the Type of Dietary Fat on Postprandial Fat Oxidation Rates: Monounsaturated (Olive Oil) vs. Saturated Fat (Cream)," *International Journal of Obesity and Related Metabolic Disorders*, 26, no. 6 (2002):814–21.

Chapter 4

1. Doreen Virtue, *Constant Craving A–Z* (Carlsbad, CA: Hay House, 1999).
2. Jennifer A. Linde, Robert W. Jeffery, Simone A. French, Nicolaas P. Pronk, Raymond G. Boyle, "Self-Weighing in Weight Gain Prevention and Weight Loss Trials," *Annals of Behavioral Medicine*, 30, no. 3 (2005):210–16.
3. http://www.foodandmood.org/Pages/sh-survey.html
4. Mikko Laaksonen, Sirpa Sarlio-Lähteenkorva, Päivi Leino-Arjas, Pekka Martikainen, and Eero Lahelma, "Body Weight and Health Status: Importance of Socioeconomic Position and Working Conditions," *Obesity Research*, 13 (2005):2169–77.
5. Jos A. Bosch, Eco J.C. de Geus, Angele Kelder, Enno C.I. Veerman, Johan Hoogstraten, and Arie V. Nieuw Amerongen, "Differential Effects of Active versus Passive Coping on Secretory Immunity," *Psychophysiology*, 38, no. 5 (2001), doi:10.1111/1469–8986.3850836.
6. Ann Hettinger, "Rest Assured," *Prevention*, 59, no. 12 (December 2007):48.
7. Ann Hettinger, "Rest Assured," *Prevention*, 59, no. 12 (December 2007):48.
8. D.L. Sherrill, K. Kotchou, S.F. Quan, "Association of Physical Activity and Human Sleep Disorders," *Archives of Internal Medicine*, 158, no. 17 (September 28, 1998):1894–98, http://archinte.ama-assn.org/cgi/reprint/158/17/1894.

Chapter 5

1. Philip S. Chua, "Air Travel: Medical Tips," *Heart to Heart Talk, CEBU Cardiovascular Center*, (2003), http://www.cebudoctorsuniversity.edu/hospital/cardio/chua2.html.
2. J.W. Pennebaker, J.K. Kiecolt-Glaser, and R. Glaser, "Disclosure of Traumas and Immune Function: Health Implications for Psychotherapy," *Journal of Consulting and Clinical Psychology*, 56 (1988):239–45.

Chapter 7

1. Steven Reinberg, "Excess Pounds Raise Women's Cancer Risk," *HealthDay* (November 7, 2007), http://body.aol.com/condition-center/breast-cancer/news/article/_a/excess-pounds-raise-womens-cancer-risk/n20071107090309990041.

Chapter 10

1. I. Giannopoulou, L.L. Ploutz-Snyder, R. Carhart, R.S. Weinstock, B. Fernhall, S. Goulopoulou, and J.A. Kanaley, "Exercise Is Required for Visceral Fat Loss in Postmenopausal Women with Type 2 Diabetes," *Journal of Clinical Endocrinology & Metabolism*, 90, no. 3 (2005):1511–18.

2. S.K. Park, J.H. Park, Y.C. Kwon, H.S. Kim, M.S. Yoon, and H.T. Park, "The Effect of Combined Aerobic and Resistance Exercise Training on Abdominal Fat in Obese Middle-Aged Women," *Journal of Physiological Anthropology and Applied Human Science*, 22, no. 3 (May 2003):129–35.

3. Melinda L. Irwin, Yutaka Yasui, Cornelia M. Ulrich, Deborah Bowen, Rebecca E. Rudolph, Robert S. Schwartz, Michi Yukawa, Erin Aiello, John D. Potter, and Anne McTiernan, "Effect of Exercise on Total and Intra-abdominal Body Fat in Postmenopausal Women," *JAMA*, 289 (2003):323–30.

4. "Depression and Anxiety: Exercise Eases Symptoms," *MayoClinic.com* (October 23, 2006), http://www.mayoclinic.com/health/depression-and-exercise/MH00043.

5. Anne J. Blood and Robert J. Zatorre, "Intensely Pleasurable Responses to Music Correlate with Activity in Brain Regions Implicated in Reward and Emotion," *Proceedings of the National Academy of Sciences*, 98, no. 20 (September 25, 2001): 11818–23.

6. Charles F. Emery, Evana T. Hsiao, Scott M. Hill, and David J. Frid, "Short-Term Effects of Exercise and Music on Cognitive Performance among Participants in a Cardiac Rehabilitation Program," *Heart & Lung: The Journal of Acute and Critical Care*, 32, issue 6 (November/December 2003):368–73.

Chapter 11

1. "With Obesity on the Rise, Dieting a Constant Concern," *Calorie Control*, 29 (Fall 2007), http://www.caloriecontrol.org/pdf/ccc%20comm%20fall07_3.pdf.

2. Willard Bishop, "Making Healthy Eating Easier," *Shopping for Health 2006*, survey by *Prevention* magazine (2006).

3. M.L. Irwin, Y. Yasui, C.M. Ulrich, D. Bowen, R.E. Rudolph, R.S. Schwartz, M. Yukawa, E. Aiello, J.D. Potter, A. McTiernan, "Effect of Exercise on Total and Intra-abdominal Body Fat in Postmenopausal Women: A Randomized Controlled Trial," *JAMA*, 289, no. 3 (January 15, 2003):323–30, http://jama.ama-assn.org/cgi/content/full/289/3/323?ijkey=2ffd96d981677fb09007213e18cda542e6ed4cc0.

index

Boldface page references indicate photographs.

Underscored references indicate boxed text and tables.

Lose up to 11 inches of body fat in 32 days!

INTRODUCING
flatbellydiet.com!

Finally, the editors of *Prevention* have developed a science-based diet that directly targets harmful belly fat! Lose up to 15 pounds while you slash your risk of heart disease, stroke, and type 2 diabetes. Here's just a sampling of what you'll get by signing up for the **FLAT BELLY DIET** online.

- **Easy-to-Use Food Logs and Meal Plans**
- **Access to Expert Help**
- **Daily Video Inspiration and Tips**
- **Community Support**

SIGN UP TODAY FOR YOUR 30-DAY RISK-FREE TRIAL AT:

flatbellydiet.com/bookoffer

200981601

FIRM UP FAST WITH
PREVENTION FITNESS DVDs.

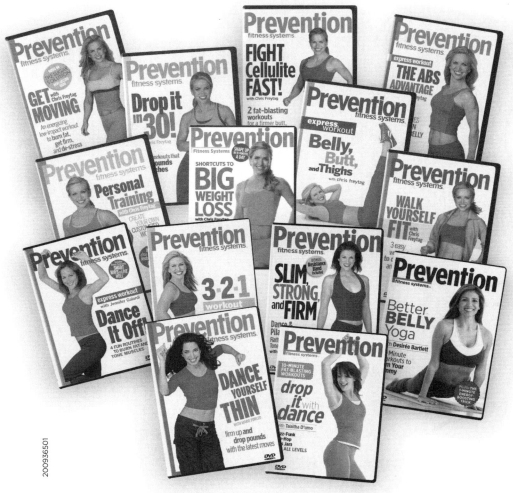

No matter what your goal, from building better cardiovascular health to shedding excess pounds, odds are Prevention Fitness Systems has an easy-to-follow DVD to help you achieve it. And since each has been designed by the fitness editors of *Prevention* magazine, you know that they're safe, effective, and made with your total health in mind.

AVAILABLE IN STORES NOW!
www.prevention.com/shop